AEP

9/30/10

$4.07

Caring for Difficult Patients

A Guide for Nursing Professionals

by Dr. Joseph Koob

B. Mus., M.A., M.S., Ed.D.

with Dr. Pam Koob

PhD, APRN, BC

ISBN 0-7414-3768-6

For more information address inquiries to NEJS Publications, Box 32, Saline, MI, 48176, or visit or e-mail

business2@difficultpeople.org

A difficultpeople.org publication

Published by:

INFI∞ITY
PUBLISHING.COM

1094 New DeHaven Street, Suite 100
West Conshohocken, PA 19428-2713
Info@buybooksontheweb.com
www.buybooksontheweb.com
Toll-free (877) BUY BOOK
Local Phone (610) 941-9999
Fax (610) 941-9959

Printed in the United States of America

Printed on Recycled Paper

Published March 2007

Table of Contents

Preface

Professionalism and Caring

I believe that the Nursing profession is one of the most admired in America. We think of Nurses as being professional. That is, they have a knowledge base and skill set that is unique and valued and that the quality of their work is important to them. We also, very importantly, think of Nurses as people who care about their patients – they are concerned with our well-being when we are under their care. These considerations are the focal point for our discussion on how to best deal with difficult patients.

This book will specifically consider the concerns that arise when Nurses encounter patients who are difficult. While we will very briefly consider other important relationships Nurses have in the work place – their peers, Nursing Supervisors, and Physicians – the emphasis here will be on the unique relationship that develops when a Nurse interacts with a client, a patient.

This is a key consideration. A patient, either directly or indirectly, is a customer. A Nurse is the service provider. As such, certain parameters are automatically set up that create general guidelines for action. The customer expects to be treated in a certain way; the Nurse is expected to provide a certain type of service. Boundaries, whether written or tacit, are drawn as a result. Both the Nurse and the patient are expected to interact appropriately and considerately within those parameters.

Patients/customers expect you, the Nurse, to be professional; and in a sense that is far more important than most other service professions, they expect you to care. The focus of this book is to demonstrate how you, the Nursing professional, can use these two key concepts – professionalism and caring – to

i

your advantage and to the patient's advantage in dealing with difficult concerns.

Yes, there will always be difficult people we have to deal with both professionally and non-professionally. While I am not a Nurse, I have written many books about "Understanding and Working with Difficult People and in Difficult Situations." I do have an intimate knowledge of the Nursing profession from Nursing professionals, research, and study. Dr. Pam Koob, whose input has been invaluable to the writing of this book, is a consummate Nursing Professional with years of caring experience at all levels of Nursing and in many different hands-on experiential situations. Her work experience includes, but is not limited to: general care, Nurse Practitioner, ER, Hospital, University-level teaching, and Wound Care Nursing.

Note: Dr. J. Koob's books, *Succeeding with Difficult Coworkers*, *Succeeding with Difficult Bosses*, and *Dealing with Difficult Customers*, all have detailed considerations in working with these specific types of relationships and concerns.

Addendum

Nurses/Nursing and Physicians will be capitalized throughout this text as a respectful gesture to two quality service professions.

Use of gender: I typically use gender indiscriminately. Men and women can be equally difficult and I make every effort to avoid assigning characteristics to one gender or another.

Approaching this book

As a long time educator and author of educational materials I try to organize information in the most easily accessible manner for everyone. As you will see, this book presents concepts in a broad outline fashion that serves to emphasize Key Ideas and Terminology. Materials are presented in sections and sub-sections that are laid out to emphasize relationships between major points, definitions and explanations, as well as knowledge, understandings, skills, and tools. Optional exercises and provocative questions are provided at the end of each Chapter as a means to extend your personal growth and understanding of the ideas presented.

Thanks

My Special Thanks to Pam Koob, my stepmother and co-author; my readers – Lisa, my beautiful wife; Anne Duston, editor extraordinaire; Allison Gold, R.N., M.A.; Amy Arneric, R.N., B.S.N.; Nathan, my son and graduate English major, for their help with this project.

Part I

Introduction

"The delivery of high quality care depends increasingly on 'processing skills' (communication, empathy, willingness to listen, common goals, ability to find alternative ways of solving problems, etc.) in addition to 'medical/care competence."

(Skjorshammer, Scandinavian J Caring Sci, 1999)

Chapter 1

Key Ideas

TLC

Author's Note: I truly believe that the phrase Tender Loving Care is how **the patient**, and this is a key point, sees the Nursing profession. However you, as a professional, consider or interpret this, it is important to always keep in mind what patients think and expect. Patients not only expect you to be a consummate professional, they expect you to care – something that can be interpreted in a variety of ways:

To give them quality Nursing care

To care about how they feel, what they think, who they are

To care about making them 'better'

To care that they are a fellow human being and you are intimately involved with their well-being for this moment in time

In some ways this is a heavy 'extra' burden that is placed on your profession. How you approach this expectation, especially with difficult patients, can make all the difference in how that patient behaves, reacts, acts, and generally deals with you and others involved with his/her care.

How you as a professional handle this important **preconception** of patients is a major emphasis in this book (see Chapter 2 and Part II, Chapters 6-9).

Professionalism

Nursing is a service profession. Patients see you as a professional and they expect you to act in a professional and caring manner.

In a sense that is almost an oxymoron. How can you be expected to be completely professional, do an outstanding job, and yet balance on that delicate thread of propriety and come across as caring as well?

Is it possible for you to balance the two?

Yes, it is possible. AND it is essential if you wish to be acknowledged as the best in a quality profession, and if you expect to be able to handle those 'difficult' cases.

Consider this: your professionalism, i.e. the high quality image you bring to your patients via your knowledge, skills, and Nursing care, sets the stage for their accepting you as a person as well, but it doesn't get you the whole way – that takes caring.

Fear

Always – and while this is an all-encompassing term it is still used here – **always** a patient feels angst when in a medical care situation, i.e., hospital, Physician's office, treatment center, etc.

Be sure to keep this key idea in mind throughout this book and at any time when you are dealing directly with a concerning situation.

Fear lies at the root of all difficult behavior.

(Perkins; Koob)

Understanding Your Approach

How you act, react, and approach a patient often dictates how they will act with/toward you. Knowing Yourself is one of the primary tools we can bring to working through difficult people concerns. ['Self-Awareness' is the first of the "Seven Keys to Being Successful with Difficult People" (Kooh, J.); See Chapter 7 and Appendix I]

The better you come to understand your affect on others and the better you begin to see how others affect you, the more control, Self-Control, you will have. This is especially important in working with difficult individuals.

[Self-Control is one of the "Seven Keys to Being Successful with Difficult People"]

Understand the Patient

First and foremost patients want you to understand how they feel.

They also want to be understood. They want you to listen to them, even if you have heard it a hundred times before, and they want to know that you have heard them. They expect you to respond in some way directly to their concerns, questions, ideas, etc.

How you feel about Yourself

Your Self-Value (Self-worth*) comes from knowing yourself and being on top of how you feel and what you think **all the time** when you are interacting with others (Self-Awareness). How you feel about yourself will have a marked impact on your patients and how they react to you.

*[Self-Worth and Self-awareness are two of the "Seven Keys to Being Successful with Difficult People"]

Communications

Nurses need to be great listeners and they need to be effective communicators. Simply put – if you communicate effectively AND caringly with your patients, you should have very few difficulties arise. Even when you do run into the inveterate complainer or ultimate sourpuss, your skills can make a major difference in any case.

Most of us know good, basic communication skills. Nurses are generally pretty good communicators and have developed approaches that work with most patients. The understanding we will emphasize in this book will be how to communicate in difficult circumstances and with difficult people – "Over-the-top Communications." These skills go beyond just good basic communications. They can be applied to all difficult people concerns at work, even those that may involve your supervisor, fellow coworkers, employees, and Physicians.

[Part III of this book, Chapters 10-14 are on 'Over-the-top' Communication skills. Also, see Chapters 21-23 – "Dealing with Families and Loved Ones," "Working with Physicians," and "Coworkers."]

Difficult Patients?

A difficult person: Any person who causes anyone else angst. (*Understanding and Working with Difficult People*, Koob. J.)

Are there many difficult patients?

You bet. It is even likely you will run into some on a fairly regular basis if you are a Nurse. There are a variety of reasons for this:

You usually see a lot of people in the course of a week, month, year (there are some in every bunch!)

Patients are afraid, often much more than they would like to admit. Fear can and does create difficult behavior in spite of how someone may normally behave.

Patients are often hurting in one way or another, usually multiple ways: physically, mentally, emotionally, and spiritually.

Patients are most often in an environment that is 'uncomfortable' at best, and often downright frightening to them. While the 'antiseptic' nature of Physicians' offices or a hospital room may be comforting on the one hand, it also sets that space out as being 'different' from what is normal. That is why delivery rooms, for example, were made more homelike in the not too distant past.

Everything you do and say within a patient's purview, and everything that you do that impacts their care, makes a difference in how they will respond to you!

Hint: It is worth thinking about this statement a lot!!!

Treat yourself well

YOU have a huge influence on others' lives. When you feel good about yourself, you will likely make a positive impression and you will have fewer difficulties even with patients who tend to be difficult. If you don't feel good about yourself, take some time and get the help you need to 'make yourself better.' It really will make a difference in how you can control and effectively deal with difficult situations and difficult people.

Questions and Ideas for Contemplation

These Key Ideas will be discussed in more detail throughout this text. Use this Chapter as a reference point and review of important concepts.

A helpful exercise is to consider each of these ideas within the context of your own work life. Write out thoughts you have and then keep them handy as you read through the rest of this book. Keep a running log and you will generate a valuable document that you can refer back to as you continue your work.

NOTE: There is an extensive Bibliography of 'Difficult People' Materials at the end of this book. Reading a wide range of materials can enhance your understanding as you develop your expertise in this area. All of Dr. Joseph Koob's books are available at www.difficultpeople.org.

Chapter 2

Tender Loving Care

"Ultimately we all want to be cared for, understood, treated well, and appreciated.

It may not seem that is what a person who is currently being obnoxious, rude, and/or pervasively negative really wants, but if you take off enough layers, you'll get there."

(Koob, J.)

CARING

Pam Koob, PhD, APRN, BC

Caring is a core value in nursing

It is a vital component of the nursing process and is now viewed as essential to the scientific process of nursing. As such it helps form the philosophical basis of nursing practice. Benner and Wrubel (1989) discussed caring as the "...most basic mode of being..."

"Caring means that people, interpersonal concerns, and things matter"

(Benner and Wrubel, p.1).

Tanner (1990) believes that caring promotes understanding by the nurse and facilitates acting on those concerns and issues important to those they care about. In her dissertation (1996), Dr Pam Koob defined caring as being fully present with patients and having positive regard for patients.

Caring is the most important function of nursing.

Caring means being honest and open with patients, as well as with colleagues.

Genuine caring requires that the nurse recognize her power and share it with her patients and colleagues.

Having meaningful experiences that involve caring as a part of your practice is what keeps us in nursing – although at times it can be a burden, it can be painful, and it can create dilemmas. As caring individuals, nurses take on "extra" if they truly exemplify caring. It is work! It can mean more stress. It does mean being involved and fully immersed in your patient's situation, including all that he brings with him to the hospital or office.

Caring requires not only involvement with your patients, but also their families and significant others.

To be a successful nursing professional, you cannot be detached and objective at all times. Caring encompasses a connectedness with your patients: A key reason why Nurses are the most highly regarded and trusted professionals in this country today is because they are perceived by the public as CARING professionals.

If you, as a Nursing professional don't truly care for and about your patients, you will never be happy in the nursing profession.

Caring is risky but worth it!

Caring for Yourself

It is important for Nurses to also take care of themselves, which can often be extremely difficult. Caring for self may mean cutting hours, changing the area where you work, or even giving up a managerial or administrative job. If we don't care for ourselves, who will? Being a truly caring Nurse is work and work is hard, so you must put yourself first so that you can BE THERE for your patients, family, friends, and colleagues. (See Chapter 25, "Taking Care of Yourself")

To be truly caring, you must take care of YOU!

Koob, P.B., *The Curriculum Revolution in Practice: A Heideggeruan Hermeneutical Analysis of the Lived Experience of Women Nurse Educators. Dissertation*, 1996.

Caring for Others

Nursing is a CARING profession. This is the most important key to understanding and working well with patients, and especially fundamental in working with difficult patients.

This perspective is so critical because it is first and foremost **the most important thing the patient expects from you**.

While you may feel that professionalism – your knowledge, the skills and tools you bring to your profession, and your professional bearing and integrity are the most critical factors to being a top quality Nurse for the patient (see next Chapter) – it is how you approach them, how they see you and **how you make them feel** that carries much more weight.

This is so important to your being 'the best you can be' that I feel adamant about the following statement:

If you can't CARE for your patients, find another profession.

If for no other reason, then you are going to find yourself dealing with lots of difficult patients.

What does TLC mean?

There are various ways to consider this phrase. However, what a patient needs and expects, more than anything else, is consideration for how they feel. The best way to give that without crossing any professional lines is to let them know you are concerned about:

Their well-being

How they feel

Understanding them

Making every effort to give them your best care

Author's Note: I have known many Nurses – I have worked with some, been friends with others, and been treated by enough in a wide variety of situations to know that there is something special about the ones who make that little bit of extra effort to care for and truly support their patients. It can be manifested in many ways, but more than anything else it is about having a caring attitude.

People can tell!

Keep in mind this key idea throughout this book, too. It is worth reiterating several times:

Everything you do and say within a patient's purview
(and their family's purview)
sets the stage for how they feel about you as a caring professional
*
EVERYTHING!

Caring

How do you show caring, real caring, without stepping over boundaries that are taboo and could be detrimental to you and/or the patient?

Caring for others enriches our lives and when they feel that from us, it enriches their lives. There is a ripple-effect that makes all of our lives that much better. Yes, there are boundaries which should not be crossed, but isn't it better to share a tear, or a joy, or a triumph, or even a lost battle with someone, than to close off your true self to them and create a distant, 'professional' only, relationship?

A good friend of mine who is a Nurse Who I have seen 'in action' on any number of occasions, has this quality. I would not describe her as overly outgoing, 'touchy-feely,' or overly emotional. She is definitely professional in both appearance and approach. But when she is with patients there is a certain quality, a focus, an intent, something that says, "I'm here for you, right now, at this moment, and how you feel is important to me." It also says, "If you are in pain, I will understand that and try to help." "If I can help you assuage your concerns in whatever ways that I can, and help you to heal, I will share your joy, as well."

This type of approach doesn't cross any patient/professional boundaries. It makes you human and in the medical profession we need people who can share their humanity.

That's TLC in a nutshell.

Are you a little bit vulnerable? Yes, but isn't it worth it?

Can you deal with it? Of course, you are a professional.

Does it matter? So much more than you might think toward helping people back to health.

Important: It also matters a tremendous amount in how patients eventually treat you and others while they are in your care.

Also – Keep in mind this important point when working with patients -- How we feel **always** impacts others.

Do you have to be careful about boundaries?

Yes, but if you are professional, you will know where those lines are and you will make sure your patients understand that fundamentally you are both caring and professional.

How can you help them to feel better AND cared for?

In Part II of this book we will discuss how you can 'ramp up' TLC so that you will have all the skills and tools you need to be successful in difficult situations.

Quality Care

Patients also expect you to offer good basic care. Your training as a Nursing professional, as well as the many things you learn on the job, are very important to how they perceive this. But there is also a more intangible element, which comes across in a variety of ways. Part of that is your professionalism and approach (Chapters 3 and 5). Another big part is how you communicate with them (Part III, Chapters 10 through 14), and most significantly, perhaps, is your ability to understand the patient and where they are coming from (Chapter 9).

You may be the best skilled Nurse in the hospital –

You may be kind, caring, compassionate, and focused on them –

You may be professional and knowledgeable –

HOWEVER – if you don't understand who this specific patient is and what is important to them, you are flinging arrows at a target with your eyes closed.

Keep this key point in mind: care is manifested in a wide variety of ways. One thing that we often forget to pay much attention to is our ability and willingness:

to help the patient understand the whole gamut of information that <u>they</u> need to help them feel cared for.

This is why communication skills are so critical.
(See Chapters 10-14)

Even with patients who have limited understanding, i.e. children, enfeebled adults, mentally and emotionally affected patients, and others, it is far better to err on the side of over-communicating, than under-communicating those key messages that say,

"I understand you are scared,"

"I understand you are hurting,"

"I will do this, this, and this to help."

[Communicating Information is an important area for Nurses and Physicians that we will address in Chapter 11).

Questions and Ideas for Contemplation

How do you care? AND How do you care for your patients?

In other words, what qualities and what approach do you bring into patient situations that says, "I am here for you?"

A key exercise: observe the Nursing professionals and Physicians you most admire. What is it about their personalities and approach that is successful with patients?

Do the same exercise observing professionals who you feel don't interact well with patients: What is it about their approach that doesn't work? What are things to avoid? What puts patients (and you) off?

The final step is to observe yourself: can you step back in your mind and see how different things you do and say effect a given response from a patient, good or bad? **Self-awareness**, Chapter 7, is fundamental to being the consummate professional.

Addendum

"So powerful is the notion of time/task imperatives in the Nurses' psyche that patients are sometimes seen as tasks, not people." *Journal of Advanced Nursing* Farrell, 35(1), 26-33, 2001

This is good point of discussion in contrast to the ideas and caring approach that has been proffered in this Chapter.

Chapter 3

Professionalism

Being a Professional

The Nurse as a professional has already been defined in two slightly different ways:

> You 'have a knowledge base and skill set that is unique and valued, and the quality of (your) work is important to you'

> You bring to patients your knowledge, skills, and Nursing care

When you graduate from a Nursing program and receive credentials to work, you are given, in effect, something that says you are now qualified to work as a Nurse. However – and this is an important element for all professionals to consider – once you take a job, and walk through that door the first day, you also have accepted professional responsibility. Responsibility that means your education has just started, and you have something to live up to.

A Profession is an ongoing commitment to quality and a continuous personal integrity associated with that profession and your work in that profession. Day one on the job is the day you really start to learn what being a Nurse is all about.

Professionals care about the quality of work they do. Professional Nurses care about the quality of care they provide – always.

In order to provide the best care during your years of tenure as a Nurse consider the following:

> It is an every day, every minute type of job. It can be quite demanding.

> You have to be open to learning new things every day for your entire career.

You learn from:

> Other coworkers/Nurses
>
> Supervisors
>
> Physicians
>
> Patients
>
> Continuing Education
>
> Professional Societies and Journals
>
> Anything and anyone that influences your professional life

It CAN be a matter of life and death.

It is ALWAYS a matter of how people feel (You, your patients, your fellow workers, etc.)

Acting Professional

When we are in any situation where we deal with, work with, or are the client of someone, what is it that makes us think that "they are a professional"?

It is not just their knowledge and skill, though these are very important, it is also some less tangible things:

> How they carry themselves
>
> How they approach us (See Chapter 5)
>
> Their confidence and control
>
> Their ability to communicate their professionalism:
>
> > both indirectly through how they do and say things
> >
> > AND
> >
> > directly through their communications and willingness to communicate with us
> >
> > (See Part III, "Communication")

Making a real difference: Learning to be the best

I have been an educator most of my life. I believe in learning. I believe that we can learn from every single situation we are in: good, bad, and neutral, IF we pay attention and don't let our egos get in the way.

For example:

You can learn a tremendous amount from a colleague who has been around the block a few times, even if she/he is a curmudgeon.

You can learn a ton from patients if you are willing to listen. Valuable information from patients is, unfortunately, sometimes ignored by health care professionals.

> Here's a hint: while patients are not generally knowledgeable about the medical field, they have the best information available about how they feel and what is affecting them. Plus, paying attention to them helps them feel like you care.

You can also learn from all those difficult patients. You can learn a great deal about how to be successful with them, by paying attention, and by using some of the skills and ideas presented in this book. You can also learn "How not to" – How not to behave; How not to treat others, and so on.

You can learn from Supervisors, Physicians, and all other medical and staff personnel, even the difficult, bossy ones, e.g., one thing you can learn is how not to be difficult and bossy!

We all have things we can teach each other. Some people are open to continual learning, some are not. A true professional never closes those gates to learning, and makes every effort to keep them wide open whenever they are at work.

Questions and Ideas for Contemplation

What does it mean, specifically, to you to be a professional? Delineating these ideas on paper can give you a foundation upon which to build your approach with patients [See Chapter 5 and also Communication Chapters 10-14]

The best way to understand this is to write down the things you admire most about your profession, the professionals you see as top-notch, and most importantly, those qualities and values you would like in yourself. A good way to think of this is: "How would I like my patients, my coworkers, my supervisor(s), and other medical professionals to see me?"

Chapter 4

Fear

Fear is at the Root of All Difficult Behavior

(Koob)

"There are only two emotions – love and fear –
and you are perpetually feeding either one or the other."

(Perkins)

Dealing with Negativity

If one accepts the premise above by Betty Perkins, that fear is in essence the root of all negative emotions, (from her book *Lion Taming: The Courage to Deal with Difficult People Including Yourself*) then any negativity we experience from others AND in ourselves comes from fear.

This is not an easy concept to wrap one's mind around, much less buy into; yet, if you take the time to think about it in any depth, it is possible to understand its feasibility. Take any 'difficult' behavior that you may encounter in your work (and life), then consider what may be driving that behavior – if you get deep enough, you'll probably find fear, angst, upset, turmoil. For example:

Rudeness

Curmudgeonly behavior

Defensiveness

Harassment

Yelling, Screaming, Foul-language

Anger

Vindictiveness

Whining, Complaining

Fight or Flight behaviors (which tend to be all-inclusive of negative 'reactive behaviors')

And so on

Actions and Reactions

Not only is it important to understand that fear is at the root of the difficult behaviors (actions) that patients present, but **our** reactions, if negative, are also rooted in fear and those reactions can, and most often do help perpetrate the negative behavior of the patient, and may likely escalate it.

What you Choose

You have choices in how you react to negativity. You can choose to stay within your calm, caring, professionalism, or you can choose something else, less positive.

Here is a very key point in working with difficult patients:

> If you can stay within yourself, i.e. that caring professional you have considered the 'fundamental **you**' at work, you will have far fewer difficulties and especially, recurring difficulties, with patients. [See Exercises at end of Chapters 3 and 4]

And the opposite is also true:

> If you react in any way negatively, even simply being defensive, you are literally setting the stage for more difficulties from this patient.

A big part of establishing a foundation from which to be successful with difficult people is to know yourself better, (See Chapter 7, "Self-Awareness). Part of that is knowing what things 'set you off,' get you upset, i.e. what, more specifically, this patient says and does that is moving you from in-control positivity to out-of-control negativity. All negative behavior we feel and exhibit means we are losing control of our true self – our professionalism, our ability to remain calm, cool, and collected, and most importantly, our caring approach.

Important: You don't have to put up with difficult or harassing behavior from patients. You have a right to stand up for yourself professionally and personally and to take care of yourself. But, there are always positive and neutral ways you can do this. The key idea here is that if you stay positive/neutral you will have much less difficult behavior in the long run; which brings us to another key point, which is the focus of the rest of this Chapter:

> When you understand that a difficult patient is anxious and stressed, and that their difficulty is rooted in fear, you can bring a more understanding approach, which can help mitigate their behavior.

Understanding Difficulties

Patients want to be understood. It can pay big dividends if you make an effort to:

> Understand that their difficult behavior is rooted in anxiety and fear

> Show them that you are concerned about how they feel

> Let them know that you will do everything in your power to help alleviate their concerns

> Make an effort to understand their concerns, their perspective, who they are as a person

> Be willing to share with them the information they need to feel more at ease with the situation

> Communicate all of the above to/with them

Making the effort to understand the difficulties a patient faces changes your perspective and approach. That will affect the patient's behavior toward you and, importantly, it gives you the opportunity to step back and see their behavior in a different light.

Think about how the following are different:

> You enter a patient's room. They start swearing at you, complaining that you and the Physicians are incompetent, this hospital is a junk heap, and on and on. They resist everything you try to do, and in spite of your professionalism and attempt to help them, they continue

21

to be 'impossible.'

You feel upset, eventually angry. You have a stern look; or perhaps you try to smile, but it doesn't quite happen. As professionally as possible you go about your duties in spite of the patient's behavior. [You do nothing to irritate the patient further, or to exacerbate the situation. Still, it doesn't improve.]

Time warp:

Same situation, but you come into the room, note the difficult behavior, and realize that this patient is feeling upset, fearful (probably subconsciously), and not understood.

Instead of reacting, you make an effort to further understand their upset: "Sir, sir, I can see you are upset. I am here to help. Please tell me what I can do for you that will make this situation better for you..." [and so on.]

Making an effort to understand, showing it, and verbalizing it can make all the difference in the world. If you continue along the same lines, you will likely get on top of this concern rapidly and you will have maintained your professional demeanor to boot. Not to mention the fact that you will feel much better having done so.

We will detail other similar types of interactions throughout this text, and suggest many approach skills and communication techniques THAT WORK. The key is in…

How the patient sees you

i.e., their perception of you as a caring person and as a professional Nurse.

Hint: Perceptions ARE everything. It doesn't really matter 'what IS,'

it matters what the patient <u>thinks</u> 'IS.'

"The cure for overcoming fear in people involves empowering them,"

(Perkins)

When we listen, make an effort to understand, and show that we care – we give another person the opportunity to gain some control or perceived control in a situation. It doesn't cost us anything, except perhaps to swallow a little bit of pride and ego, and it can make all the difference in how difficult a person continues to be.

Questions and Ideas for Contemplation

Try this exercise:

Think back on an encounter you have had with a difficult patient. Review and detail everything that happened:

> What about their behavior bothered you – and others

> What exactly did they say and do that created concerns – include as much detail as possible, i.e. facial expressions, gestures, tone of voice, resistance, and so on

> How you approached them – what you said and did

> How you think they felt when all was said and done – about you, about their care, about your facility and other personnel, etc

> How you felt – detail your emotional reactions, when working with them, as well as immediately following the encounter

> How you feel now, revisiting this

Keep this handy. It will be worth going through several times as you read this book. You will discover many other approaches, skills, and tools, you can use as your understanding grows.

Chapter 5

Your Approach

Everything we do and say within the purview of the patient
impacts how they respond to us and the situation,
i.e. how difficult they are.

Professionalism, Caring, and...

How the patient sees you, from the time you enter their room, creates an image in their mind – of who you are and how you do things. We have already discussed 'approach' from the important perspective of your professionalism and the need to be perceived as caring about the patient and their concerns. In this Chapter we will discuss more specific aspects of patient understanding that do relate back to these two core concepts, but also that point toward ideas that will be discussed in the next three main sections of this book: Part II, Beyond TLC; Part III Communications; and Part IV, Succeeding with Difficult Patients.

First Impressions

These are things a patient may notice when you first work with them:

> How you look
>
> How you carry yourself
>
> Your facial expression(s)
>
> Gestures and other non-verbal clues
>
> Your verbalizations
>
> How you go about your job:
>
>> Taking care of them
>>
>> Handling diagnostic tests

Doing or helping with procedures

[Author's Note: See end of this Chapter for a humorous perspective re. 'Procedures' I wrote some time ago.]

Giving medications

Etc.

How you leave them

Do you know?

How much of a handle do you have on how you perform in the key areas listed above? While what you do, how you do it, what you say, and the way you say it may work well with non-disruptive patients, our ability to understand how we come across to others can significantly improve how we succeed with patients who are 'over the edge.'

How you look

A key professional element: In professions like Nursing there are 'accepted' parameters for: what you wear; how neat and clean your appearance is; even such things as how you do your hair and what shape it is in and whether you have extraneous mementoes that take away from how a patient sees you – jewelry, etc. In a sense there is an accepted dress code.

> [Author's note: As a college professor I used to often smile inwardly when some scruffy, long-haired, ring-nosed, earring-laden, unshaved college student would get up to make a presentation or to perform. I would say to myself, 'That will change dramatically within a year of their graduation!'' Invariably after they graduated and 'came back' they had adopted a much more professional appearance – you don't get a job, otherwise. In some ways you just have to 'be your profession.']

Let's face it right up front: it is important that you look professional. Patients expect a Nurse to look pretty much top-notch at all times. Anything less than that and doubt and anxiety may creep into the equation. Therefore it is always a good idea to 'keep up appearances.' Change your uniform if it gets blood or mess on it; check your hair; adjust your clothing; and so on. Whether you 'like' to have to do this is not the issue – patients expect it.

How you carry yourself

There are fine lines between – appearing professional or being too staid; between being caring and kind, or overly gushy; and between being efficient but rigid, or competent but relaxed.

How do you appear to a patient who sees you for the first time?

Consider their situation: They may be dressed in what they often feel is a ludicrous (and embarrassing) hospital gown and sitting on the edge of a gurney when you enter the room. At the very least they are probably a bit anxious, perhaps very concerned, about how they feel and what is about to happen. If it is the first time they are seeing you, they see you as a complete stranger, which can add to their angst. All of these factors and others will affect how they perceive you.

Your best approach:

> Be confident and professional – as well as relaxed and friendly

> Focus on the patient, but keep that professionalism always present even though you will work toward establishing a caring, kind approach

> Do your job efficiently and well, but keep up your verbal communication with the patient, even if it is simply friendly banter as you work with them and their concerns

Catherine Lein suggests that as a means of self-support, take a moment to "Stop, Breathe, and Focus," before entering a patient's room. [Presentation, American Academy of Nurse Practitioners, Dallas, 2006]

Facial expressions, gestures, and other non-verbal clues

One way you can add a good bit of flexibility in your work with different (and difficult) patients is to self-observe how subtle changes in your approach affect a given situation. Some patients may respond to friendliness, a quick smile, non-threatening/caring touch, and so on. Others may actually prefer you to have a more professional, efficient, 'get-straight-to-the-problem' approach. Try different things.

Here are two key ideas – if you keep these in mind and work with them, they can make a huge difference in how patients perceive you:

> Know how what you do and say affects a patient through self-observation – over time you will build a repertoire of knowledge and skills to use

> Develop the ability to adjust as you observe the patient's reactions to you on a moment by moment basis

These ideas require some key skills:

> Knowing yourself through self-awareness (see Chapter 7)

> Understanding your patient by observing them (see Chapter 8)

> Being willing to be open and flexible when you need to be

What you say

Communications are key. Here are some preliminary ideas in prelude to Part II of this book:

> Keep up a friendly banter – be clear and calm in your vocal expression, find what seems to be a soothing, relaxing tone and cadence. This can be very effective in easing tensions, especially if you start right away and keep it going, as appropriate – again observe your patient's reaction and adjust as necessary

> Listen to your patient – make sure you understand what is important to them

> Always ask them how they feel – what are their concerns? what you can do for them? This may seem obvious, but it is not. This is often very important to how they perceive you and your concern for them

> Repeat –listen again; ask again, etc. Stay on top of the whole situation. Some patients need a good bit of

reassuring and your willingness to 'stay with' them will be appreciated.

How you Say It

Staying on top of how you say things is VERY important – inflection, tone, expression(s), stance, distancing can make a tremendous difference in how a patient 'takes' what you have said and in how they ultimately respond to you.

How you go about your job

It is definitely necessary to maintain your professionalism and do what you need to do to assist this patient. But it is also important to do it with all the considerations listed above included. Being professional, efficient, and on top of things does not have to exclude being caring, kind, and compassionate.

[Author's note: One key idea – which you can take from me, a person who has been a patient enough times, and gone through enough medical procedures – **keep the patient informed**, honestly informed, of what you are doing, and why.]

Knowledge and information are KEY to helping keep someone relaxed and accepting of what you need to accomplish. People like to be in the know even if what is happening or about to happen is not going to be so pleasant. It comes back to keeping up that friendly and informative conversation with the patient. This is especially crucial with patients who tend to be very anxious, uptight, and/or down-right curmudgeons.

Questions and Ideas for Contemplation

How do you come across?

We will visit this concept in more detail in Chapter 7, but this would be a good time to write down everything you can think of relevant to how you see yourself as you work with your patients. Self-knowledge and understanding can be very powerful tools. Once you have a handle on these you can make adjustments as needed with those 'difficult' cases.

Addendum

"Procedures"

You are sitting at the Doctor's office. Things were going fine with your annual physical until the Physician, an old family friend, suddenly turned diabolical by uttering 'THE WORD!'

"Joe, I think we need to do this PRO—CEEE---DURE."

That is when you knew life as you had known it was over. No doubt you have had enough 'PRO-CEE-DURES' to know that it almost invariably means something discomforting, if not downright painful, is about to happen to you...not to mention the embarrassment you will have to go through when this PRO-CEE-DURE is implemented in front of a room full of people (Nurses, Doctors, techs, radiologists, and anesthetists, and even possibly your significant other) AND the indisputable FACT that 99% of PRO-CEE-DURES require the insertion of something foreign into some part of your body where that something isn't naturally supposed to go AND THEN manipulating it in some way, for an extended period of time, so that the maximum discomfort and pain is achieved before the PRO-CEE-DURE is complete. AND they have the gall to say, "Just relax. This won't hurt a bit."

That's when you want to ask them if you could do it to them after they are finished.

Now wouldn't it be fun to turn the tide back on Doctors!?! The next time a Physician comes in your office, tell them that you would be glad to help, but that it requires an involved PRO-CEE-DURE. Chances are they will run the other way. They KNOW!

Well, I've got to go. I'm busy inventing PRO-CEE-DURES for the next difficult person to come into my life.

Just kidding. Have a great and hopefully PRO-CEE-DUREless day.

Best,

Joe Koob

*Weekly E-letter from Difficultpeople.org

Part II

Beyond TLC

"View your relationship with a patient as a 'Sustained Partnership' that leads to improved continuity of care."

Catherine Lein -- American Academy of Nurse Practitioners, 2006

A Caring Professional approach will make a major difference to your patients and to your success <u>with</u> patients. However, there are many subtle things you can add to the equation that can make a difference in not only how your patients see and experience you, but in how you enjoy your work and life.

Chapter 6

Kindness, Compassion, and Caring

Kindness

[Author's Note: I truly believe that kindness is one of the great attributes we can develop as human beings. On the surface it seems like something that is so simple to understand and to do, but in reality we get wrapped up in so many other things that we do forget.]

In the Nursing profession, kindness is one thing you can work on with every interaction you have, and if you do, you will have a profound affect on people over time. It is something that takes you beyond simply caring, without stepping across any boundaries between patient, professional, and staff.

Practice kindness with everyone - including yourself

Just keeping this concept firmly in our psyche as we go about our job makes a difference. It gives us that bit of energy or impulse to remember to make a difference in everyone's life.

And it is easy to do:

> What you say and how you say it
>
> Compliments and smiles bring smiles in return
>
> 'Thank you' never hurts and can mean a lot
>
> Offering to help, assist, and to go above and beyond what is 'required'
>
> Making a difference right now – with this patient – find a way
>
> Smile!

Believe it or not the general tenor of a work place affects you and everyone you interact with. When you are kind and considerate to everyone at work: staff, Physicians, supervisors, anyone there for whatever reason, you make a difference that affects you and your interactions with your patients.

> "Live your Life OUT LOUD!" (Zola, Peters, Koob)

It is almost too easy to fall back into the everyday routines and begin 'slogging' through our work week. We CAN make a difference – every day and with everyone we interact with. It is a choice we make whenever we are with someone. Choose wisely for yourself and for others.

Important Note: janitors/custodians, mail people, administrative assistants, and many others keep your life at work rolling along (or not). Kindness in all places makes a difference.

Compassion

Compassion is kindness coupled with caring. It is that one step beyond just being kind that says to someone in your care...

> you matter to me
>
> your health and well-being matter to me.

"Compassion is Kindness in action in the most difficult of circumstances"

(Koob, **Musings**)

Author's Note: There is an attitude or 'school of thought' that I, as a counselor, coach, mentor, former college professor, happen to disagree with which suggests that it can be detrimental for those of us in service professions to 'care,' 'to be compassionate,' for our clients/customers.

Here is an example of a better approach:

When my father passed away I had an airline ticket with American Airlines to fly to Oklahoma on business. Obviously that trip was put on hold and I called American to see whether I could adjust the ticket and use it at a later date. I explained the circumstances and what I hoped could be done. However, the agent told me that the ticket was a non-refundable coach fare that could not be adjusted.

The American Airline agent showed concern, understanding, kindness, and compassion. She even called in her supervisor to see if anything could be done about my request. Neither of them could help me, nor could they get past 'the rules,' but the way they dealt with me was so considerate that I simply appreciated their kindness, concern, and compassion for my circumstances. Ultimately American Airlines refunded the ticket price in full even though they couldn't 'transfer' the ticket.

From everything that transpired in that interaction I felt cared for. I felt that they genuinely understood me as a human being and were willing to open themselves up to their own feelings as a result – that is compassion!

AND, the important thing here is that it made ALL of our lives richer. It certainly didn't hurt anyone, nor was it detrimental, as far as I could tell, in any way for them or me to have shared those feelings.

If you are experiencing a major roadblock in considering these ideas – those centered around caring, kindness, and compassion – please consider the little story above carefully. Then, and I think this is one way to understand this whole consideration better, put yourself into my position and into the position of those American Airline agents.

Think about how this might affect a patient situation you have been involved in.

A difficult patient situation?

The truth is, it is the difficult patients, the ones who are hardest to reach, that need all the kindness, compassion, and caring they can get.

There are always ways we can be kind and when we add compassion to that, we are saying to ourselves and others – we all matter – and that is what makes us human.

Questions and Ideas for Contemplation

You know Nursing. Brainstorm a list of ideas, little kindnesses, that you can use throughout your place of work, and with your patients. Then put them in action every day.

You may set a ball rolling that comes back in many positive ways for you and for everyone else. A kind, open, friendly place to work in is so much better than anything else and someone has to be the catalyst. Why not you?

Chapter 7

Self -Awareness

"Know Yourself"

(Socrates)

YOU make all the difference!

Analyze any difficult situation you find yourself in and you can find reasons and excuses to blame it on someone or something else...

> And you may be right

>> And you have every right to complain and blame

>>> And 99.9% out of a 100% the situation ain't gonna get any better as a result.

Choose to be in control of who you are and how you present yourself

Choose to be on top of things

Choose to be proactive about finding a solution

Choose to be a caring professional

It is all about Paying Attention

And that starts with paying attention to yourself:

> How are you coming across?

> How is the patient reacting to what you do?

> How are you reacting to what the patient does?

>> How do you feel?

>> What are you thinking?

And paying attention includes:

> Your making an effort to understand how the patient perceives you (see below).

AND, very importantly, paying attention to...

> What you are about to do?

These are all great questions to ask yourself when you find yourself in any difficult situation with another person, because they set the stage for you to maintain your self-control and composure, which in turn gives you the platform from which to maintain and improve the circumstance.

How are you coming across?

How does the patient perceive you?

These are two related, but different questions. The first is directly related to self-observation; the second, to observing the patient's reactions and responses to you.

Being aware of how you perceive yourself as you enter into a difficult situation, and as the difficult situation unfolds, is very important. It helps you take a step back mentally and emotionally, and helps you maintain self-control. When you are in control, i.e. when the patient's poor behavior is NOT affecting how you maintain your composure, your ability to do your job professionally, and your ability to stay within your calm, caring, kind approach, you have a good chance of defusing any difficulties that may arise.

Important: difficult people expect us to react to their difficulty. While they may not understand this consciously, they are after something – to gain our attention, to get something they want, to have what they perceive to be a need filled, etc. (see next Chapter, "Understanding the Patient").

When we don't react to their negativity, their expectations are left unfulfilled and we are then capable of filling their needs, wants, and desires in more positive, life-enhancing ways.

Knowing yourself may seem like a no-brainer, but the truth is, we often do not practice self-awareness enough. It pays to get in the habit of automatically shifting gears mentally and emotionally whenever you find yourself dealing with a difficult person and/or situation. We do this by taking that little instant to step back in our mind to say, "What's going on here? How is this affecting me? How am I feeling? What do I need to do to stay on top of this? What knowledge, skills, tools do I have to help deal with this?" And so on.

If you practice self-observation, you can do this virtually instantaneously – because you don't actually have to ask yourself those questions, you become those questions. They are part of how you deal with difficulties.

Example:

A patient is being unruly and uncooperative. He complains about everything you do, and generally in terms that are uncalled for (blaming, name-calling, swear words, etc.) and even resists the things you are trying to do to assist him.

Instead of reacting to his difficult behavior, as we all typically might, by getting upset, frustrated, tense, defensive, and so on, you 'step back,' and self-observe:

> "Okay, this guy's really trying to get me to react to his negativity. I am feeling a bit tense, but I can handle it. He is trying to get me to react by calling me names and putting me down, I don't need to buy into this..."

Just this one 'step' in dealing with a difficult person changes the stage setting. By not **reacting** (out-of-control) to the negativity of another, and simply by paying attention to how we feel, and what we are thinking, we are capable of thinking through the situation (Self-awareness leads to Self-control), maintaining our self-worth and self-confidence in spite of what they do, and putting ourselves in a position to **respond** (be in control) more positively.

Know: how you feel, what you are thinking, and then add to that the understanding – "this is how I would normally react to this type of rude, inconsiderate behavior" –

> I would get upset and feel bad about myself.

> I would get angry and tense.

I would feel guilty about not handling this better.

If I really let him get to me, I would get defensive and probably get a bit stiff in my responses to him, lose my smile, become efficient, but distanced, and maybe even mechanical in my treatment.

I would carry this negative experience around with me the rest of the day.

And so on.

Important: Once you start consciously practicing self-awareness, you will get a handle on your typical reactions very quickly.

Self-awareness gives you choices. It is your most important skill in being able to deal with difficult patients and the problem situations they create.

Self-Awareness helps you build and maintain:

> **Self-Worth**

> **Self-Confidence**

> **Self-Control**

And it helps you stay within yourself so you can maintain your:

> **Honesty** (to your own fundamental professionalism and values)

> **Kindness**

> **Positivity**

[These are the **Seven Keys to Understanding and Working with Difficult People**. For a more detailed exposition on these seven key concepts see Appendix I.]

The patient

Observing how the patient sees you and how he responds to you – to what you say and do – is also an important part of the total equation. When you can mentally stay alert as to how you are coming across to a patient, you can make immediate and subtle changes to your approach that can help mitigate difficulties.

Self-awareness and self-observation are skills you need to stay on-top of the whole time you are with a patient. The more you can be tuned in to the whole situation, the better you will be able to maintain your own composure and to adjust to the patient's composure and actions.

As you work with this technique you will develop personal skills that you find work best for you. You may find that a certain gesture is calming, a way of saying something helps reduce a patient's angst, and so on. Use what works, create and be flexible when you need to be, and above all pay attention – it gives you that extra edge you need when dealing with difficult circumstances.

Questions and Ideas for Contemplation

How do you react with/to a difficult patient?

Can you envision/remember an encounter with a patient that caused you some perturbation? How did you feel? What were you thinking? What did you say and do? How did the patient react to what you did and to what you said? Write this all out in detail.

Then, try to work out in your mind how this situation might change if you stayed on top of it from the start by not reacting to the patient's negativity (in any way!) and thus gave yourself the opportunity to maintain your caring professionalism throughout. What other choices and responses might make a difference?

Chapter 8

Self-Worth

How we feel about ourselves is critical to how we are perceived by others. Your self-confident, professional approach to your patients helps them feel confident about your abilities. This Chapter is about how you feel and how that affects your interactions with others, especially difficult others.

Core values

If we make the effort to really think about who we are, each of us has a set of values that we truly believe in. These core values and qualities are what set the stage for our interactions with the rest of the world.

When you understand your core values, and bring them more to the surface you are much more likely to 'carry them with you' on a regular basis – in other words, you will become these values in your interactions with others.

How to?

> Author's Note: The exercise below is a good way to discover what we value most. I initially wrote about this for my book, "Guiding Children," and have found it so useful that I have used it in several of my other works. Take some time today to try this. You might be surprised at what you come up with. By working through this exercise you will have created something that will be of value to you for the rest of your life.

Ask yourself this question:

> "What values and qualities would I like my children to exemplify as they grow up?"

Whether you have children, or even plan to have children, is not a critical issue. What is important is that you think very specifically about how you would envision someone you are/will be responsible for as they grow up. What are the values you want them to hold dear and what are the qualities you wish they will have?

Important: stick to values and qualities, i.e. "I want my child to be honest," or "I would like my child to respect others." Try to be specific. Statements like, "I want my child to be good," or "I want my child to have good religious values," are too broad.

Keep at this until you have what you feel is a fairly comprehensive list. You can write/add as much or as little as you like, but once your list becomes finalized it is a good idea to narrow it down to the ten most important qualities you would wish them to exemplify. If you want, you can further delineate the top three and even select one value that you feel is most important.

These are probably the very core values that you wish you could exemplify in your own life. They are the ideals you hold closest to your heart.

How can you bring them to the fore?

How can you make them part of your daily life with your patients, with everyone?

You just did.

Go back often and revisit your list. Remind yourself daily, in every interaction you have with others, that this is who you truly want to be. It will help you focus your life. It will enhance your self-worth – who you are and what you are about in your life and work and in your interactions with others.

Yes, we all make mistakes. We all 'get away from' our true self at times. Sometimes we lose focus, or get affected by the negativity of others. Sometimes we are ill, or a situation threatens to overwhelm us. However, when you 'know yourself,' you know what is important for you to get back to – this gives you a solid foundation of self that you can return to as you overcome the difficulties you have been dealing with in life and at work.

What is Self-Worth?

Self worth is how we value ourselves. It is not egotism, which is placing ourselves above others. It is exemplified in our daily lives by how we approach other people and our tasks. When we feel good about who we are, what we believe in, and are able to manifest that, we have a far better chance of dealing with difficulties.

It does have to do with believing in ourselves.

It does have to do with being willing to assert or stand up for ourselves and what we believe – intelligently and kindly.

It also has to do with how we perceive and treat others – respectfully as fellow humans, regardless of their foibles, eccentricities, and despite their rude, abrasive, negatively-laden behaviors.

When you know your foundation, those values and qualities that are at your core, the difficulties of others become less key to the enjoyment and enrichment of your own life and work.

Personality

Some of us are outgoing, Type A personalities; some of us are more introverted, and some of us are down-right shy. Where are you on this spectrum? AND how does that affect your interactions with others, particularly difficult others?

> Author's Note: I fall into the more introverted type, but I have also learned to value who I am and what I believe. That gives me the inner self-confidence to deal with difficult concerns and difficult others.

Self-worth sets the stage, not for your fundamental personality, but for how you feel as you live your life.

Still feel you could use some assertiveness training and positive self-image work?

We improve our Self-Worth through Self-Awareness

Paying attention to who we are and how we interact with the

world is how we help build our self-worth and self-confidence: root yourself in the values you hold closest to your heart and then practice bringing those to the fore as you work through each day. If you keep working at it, you will be surprised at how quickly you begin to value yourself more, trust yourself more in difficult situations, and appear more confident and outgoing with others.

Try it. It is well worth the effort –

**"When you value yourself,
others will learn to value who you are, too."**

(Koob)

Questions and Ideas for Contemplation

Do the exercise above. It will be more valuable to you than you can imagine. This is not a 'set' list; it is a dynamic list and you can adjust it at any time as you continue to grow in wisdom.

When you have a fairly good list, make several copies and keep them handy. Tape one to your computer; laminate one and keep it in your wallet or purse; post one in your office. Then refer back to the 'real you' as frequently as possible – you will find that you will start bringing that 'you' more and more into your interactions with everyone.

Chapter 9

Understanding the Patient

Do you know what I need? What I want? What I desire?

Can you give these to me without compromising your integrity, professionalism, and ability to show caring and understanding?

A patient may not ask you these specific questions, but they feel them and they hope that you, the Nursing professional, understands how important they are.

Start with a key premise

As mentioned previously, **difficulty is rooted in fear** and fear (angst, upset, edginess, turmoil, tension, stress, perturbation) **is part of any clinical situation with a patient.**

Even if a patient is in your office for a positive reason – hoping her routine amniocentesis is good news for her baby; receiving confirmation that an x-ray is negative; having a physical (remember those procedures!); and so on – they will likely be ill at ease at the very least.

Your approach, demeanor, and professionalism matter!

Your ability to show the patient that you understand their concerns, needs, and desires matters a great deal.

"Be patient centered"

(Lein)

What a patient needs, wants, and desires

To receive the best of care.

To be treated kindly and courteously (even if they are not being that way themselves!)

To have your focus on them and their concerns

To be treated with respect: talked to, kept informed

To be understood

You are capable of giving all of these things in ANY circumstance, difficult or otherwise, without affecting your caring professionalism and integrity. When someone is being difficult it CAN be tough, but when you can offer what a patient needs and wants in spite of how they present themselves to you, you will assuage many of their concerns, mitigate difficulties more readily, and feel better about your own abilities as a professional as a result.

Be willing to ask what a patient needs/wants. Listen to them. Is what they want feasible? Can you provide it within ethical and care-giving boundaries?

Asking helps the patient feel they have some say in their care and it also shows concern, which in turn helps them feel more in control.

Can you work with a patient in such a way as to help them maintain their dignity, and importantly, some sense of control of the situation? Can you give them the power to provide input into what is happening, about to happen, what needs to happen – give them the chance to set personal goals within the constraints of the care that is needed? (Lein).

You can if you pay attention to them, pay attention to your communications with them, develop your skills and techniques in presenting yourself and needed information in the best possible manner: see Communication Techniques, Chapters 10-14.

Assumptions – the mother of many difficulties

When in doubt – ask!

Many, many times difficult situations escalate because people make assumptions. You are the one with the power to change the dynamics of a situation in which a patient is being difficult – often you can do that by simply being willing to ask them what they need, what they want, what they desire.

46

"Mr. Smith, what can I do to make this situation better for you?"

"Mrs. Jones, I know you are upset, please tell me what I can do to help?"

"Johnny, you look scared. Can I help you to feel better about what we are going to do here? Do you have any questions I can answer?"

Asking is a great tool:

It shows respect

It opens doors

It tells the patient that you care about what they are feeling and thinking

It moves rapidly away from negativity in many instances

It can be informative for you and for the patient

Follow-up your questions with good listening skills, and by responding to what they say and what information they give you.

Author's Note: One of the biggest frustrations I have had as a patient with Physicians and Nurses is when they seem unwilling to explain things to me. This could be because they don't want to take the time or because (and it often feels this way whether it is or not) they don't think I will understand or care. When that is the case, then as a patient, I am willing to ask.

However! And this is very important – many patients feel intimidated by their surroundings and the people who are caring for them. Physicians and Nurses are professionals. You may be a BIG DEAL to them and they may be very shy of opening up to you. Your willingness to ask about what is important to them may open up the door for them to feel brave enough to tell you how they are feeling and what they are thinking.

Unfortunately that discomfort can easily translate into difficult behavior. When Physicians and Nurses don't make the effort to understand their patients, and to take that extra step to understand by 'asking,' patients can and often do feel:

Uncared for – in spite of the good service you may provide

Less than, Not-good-enough – like they don't matter

Put-down, Guilty, Ashamed

Ignored

Frustrated, Upset, Angry

Uninformed

Important: these may be below the surface, but they will come out eventually

By being open, honest, and willing to inquire into a patient's concerns you open up many, many doors. This effort, a simple courtesy, really, can make more of a difference than just about anything else in this book toward being effective with a difficult patient. Of course, you will occasionally run into someone who doesn't respond to your best efforts, but most will.

Patient's Intent

The primary intent of any patient is two-fold:

Get healthy – in other words, find out what is wrong and get it fixed (something you may or may not be able to provide in part or in whole).

And,

To have this accomplished with the least amount of discomfort (again, something you may or may not be able to provide in part or in whole).

Because these are professionally-based results, you may be unable to always provide them, depending on the case. That is why everything written above about understanding a patient's needs, wants, and desires is so crucial – they ARE things you can almost always provide.

Questions and Ideas for Contemplation

Can you place yourself in a patient's shoes and understand the concerns they may have?

Can you step beyond their difficult behavior and see the fear they are dealing with?

Can you find ways to help mitigate their concerns by your approach, your willingness to be open to who they are and what they want?

Can you learn, and this is the tough part, not to jump to conclusions, not to make assumptions, but to be willing to ask and listen so that your patient really does feel understood and does feel that you truly care about who they are and what is important to them?

Part III

Communication

A caring, professional approach will make a major difference to your patients and to your success with patients. However, there are many subtle things you can add to this equation that can make a difference – not only in how your patients see and experience you, but in how you enjoy your work and life.

Chapter 10

Good Communication made Great

We all would like to think of ourselves as good communicators. What is actually much closer to the truth is that we all can improve our communication skills – not because we are bad communicators or because we don't know how to communicate well – but because we forget.

It is easy to let things slide when it comes to communication. This is especially easy to do at work, because we have so many other things we are involved with, and concerned about, that we can miss many opportunities to be really effective in our interactions with others.

Pay attention!

Those two words again...when we **pay attention** to ourselves and others IT MATTERS!

Patients, especially difficult patients, will often be much more amenable to who you are and what you are doing, if you are on the top of your game and if you keep the communication flowing. Pay attention to what you say, how you say it, and how the patient responds. Then you will be able to temper your interactions with them to achieve the best possible outcome. Plus they will appreciate your focus and attention.

Good basic Communication Skills

Talk – a calm, clear, soothing voice can help ease a patient's anxiety

Watch HOW you say things – any hint of negativity, sarcasm, etc. will erase any good you have done and will often exacerbate the situation. Pay attention to your tone, inflection, demeanor, expressions, etc. Be sincere and open.

Ask – them about themselves, what is important to them, etc. When you get a patient talking, they are more likely to calm down and work with, rather than against, you. Hint: almost everyone likes to talk about themselves.

Ask – them what they need, want, and desire to make this situation easier for them. Information sharing, when appropriate – and it is rare that it isn't – often helps with difficult patients. By giving them what they want – to know what is going on, how they are doing, etc., you can ease much of their angst. Important: if you don't know or can't tell them, tell them you don't know or can't tell them. Honesty is also appreciated

Talk – Keep them informed of what is going on, what is about to happen, etc. For instance – "I'm doing this, because...," "We need to do...," "This may be a bit uncomfortable...," and so on. [Again, your reassuring voice, your honest conversation, and your willingness to be open with them can and often does, help ease tensions.]

Ask – Remember: if you are in a clinic setting or any setting where you will see this patient more than once, take the time to really know some things about them. Ask them about things you can use as conversational touchstones each time they come in. People really appreciate these efforts. [For example: A curmudgeonly grandmother may share information about her kids and grandkids if you ask, and when she comes back for another visit you can always start right off with, "Marge, I remember you said that your daughter, Maggie, is an artist. What kind of medium does she work with?" And so on.]

Don't just Talk and Ask – Listen...a no-brainer, right? Yes, it should be. Unfortunately there's that 'I'm much too busy' factor that tends to get in the way.

> Listening well denotes many things to another person –
> that they are important, that you care about them, that you
> want to understand, and so on. It is respectful, and
> sometimes that is all it takes for a person to 'come
> around' and be less difficult.

Give your patient a chance to ask questions – and be willing to take time to listen carefully as the dialogue develops.

[Author's Note: My most frustrating moments with Physicians and Nurses have been when I asked a question which was then ignored; or when someone asked me something and then seemingly completely ignored what I had to say. People expect you to pay attention to everything they say – they are saying it because it is important to them.]

Which is better?

A frustrated patient who creates a good bit of angst for everyone he/she comes in contact with?

Or

Taking that extra time to 'be with' a patient and to understand their concerns?

The MOST frustrating patient experiences have at their heart poor communications by the care-givers!

Physicians/Nurses –

> who are in too much of a hurry to do anything but the
> minimum 'in and out' diagnosis, treatment, and then move
> on

> who don't communicate with their patients beyond a bare
> minimum

> who ignore a patient's concerns, complaints, feelings,
> ideas (Yes, the patient's ideas about their illness may be

way off base, but they need to understand why they are off base and they won't unless you talk with them.)

who seem unwilling to ask and/or listen

whose work ideal is rooted in professional excellence and efficiency, but lacks kindness, caring, and compassion

who fail to share information with their patients that can help ease their worries and concerns

You can avoid many patient frustrations if you open up your communications from the start. It is amazing the difference we make if we begin to pay closer attention to how we communicate, and if we are willing to open up our communications with others. This applies to everyone we interact with at work: our patients, coworkers, Physicians, supervisors, and staff.

Questions and Ideas for Contemplation

Room for improvement? Try rating yourself on your basic communication skills. Self-observe over the next week as you interact with patients and see what areas you might make some improvements in.

Take some time to see if adjustments you make seem to make a difference in how patients respond to you. You will likely be pleasantly surprised.

Chapter 11

Information

The flow of information throughout a work environment is very important to how you feel and hence, how you interact with patients. Whenever possible try to keep lines of communication open between key players:

Physicians and Patients

Coworkers and Patients

Staff and Patients

Physicians, Coworkers, and Staff

While it is great to hope that everyone will pitch in and your workplace will be an ideal network of information sharing, that is rarely the case.

Author's Note: I have found in my own work as a manager (director, Chair, Dean, etc.), executive and personal coach, and employee, that if I take the initiative and help the basic flow of information, the whole team/office will benefit.

It may take only one person on a team to set better overall communications in motion. It is worth the little bit of extra effort that it may take.

Keys to Information Sharing

- Don't assume someone understands something – if there is any doubt, ask.

- Reiterate important ideas/information – repetition IS the mother of good memory. Use it.

- Get stuff in writing/put stuff in writing – this is especially helpful for patients. As a patient I know that while I think

I will remember everything someone tells me, that is rarely the case, and when a Nurse or Physician writes it down, I have something concrete to fall back on.

- Follow-up whenever feasible – great communications and information sharing can get backlogged by any small glitch in the system. That could be a grumpy and/or stubborn patient, an over-worked supervisor, or anyone else within the information network stream. It doesn't hurt to recheck. Just be sure to do so kindly – avoiding accusations, blaming , and complaining in the process.

> Follow-up with patients! A quick phone call can mean a great deal to a patient, especially if information becomes available that is important to them and it is appropriate to share it with them. For your regular patients, or 'just because,' touching base with them can mean a great deal. (Koob, Lein)

> While this will take some time and you are probably more than busy, this is one of those extras that expresses our humanity to others. It is one of those gestures that makes the Nursing profession what it is.

- Seek specificity/Verify a patient's understanding – most patients are somewhat intimidated by Doctors and Nurses. They may never ask, even though they didn't understand anything you told them. A great tool, especially if dealing with someone who may be resisting care, or who is just out-of-sorts, is to ask them what they understood. Follow-through with a give and take until you feel you have gotten the information across successfully.

- Be specific – be willing to ask the patient for more in-depth information when they are sharing their thoughts with you. When it comes to health care, important points, even critical information, are often in the details. Find out.

- Remain open – to ideas, suggestions, feedback, and any clues that tell you how a patient (or another person) is feeling and what they are thinking. True understanding and care will happen only if you are willing to 'be available' for what a patient feels is important.

- Ask yourself: "What does this person need from me? Want from me? Am I able to provide it? If not, what can I provide and what information will help ease their concerns?" If you are willing to ask these types of questions and make an effort to answer them by being action/solution-oriented, you will have far fewer difficult patient issues throughout your interactions at work.

- Be Concise – While it is important to talk with patients and help them feel at ease and cared for, brief, to the point, effective communications that – and this is a key point – have your sincere concern for quality at the root are best when passing on information. That doesn't take volume; it takes intelligent, well-chosen, focused communications coupled with a willingness to be the catalyst to keep information flowing.

Written Information Sharing

At some point in any patient's care information needs to be written down and presented in some form to others – instructions, forms, e-mail, memos, etc. How can you be most effective in sharing written information and ensuring that others will look at it and understand it when they do?

Forms and instructions may seem intelligible to you (and or the attending physician), but may mean little to a patient unless explained in detail, or written in an easily understandable way.

E-mail has become a preferred method for sharing information, yet for many people it has become just the opposite of its potential: too many e-mails – poorly written, in confusing formats, too verbose, etc. As Nurses you also have a myriad of forms to complete, charting to do, etc.

Keep in mind that any information being transmitted in any form about a patient can ultimately affect their care whether it is something that ends up in a file, or in someone else's purview.

Key Ideas when putting something in Writing

Cover the topic/information thoroughly for the patient or receiver, but if at all possible – Keep it brief!

> The most common mistake in written communications is trying to say too much. Most people are much too busy to read a volume of material. They want to be able to consume the gist of something as quickly as possible. Practice writing terse but informative instructions, e-mails, memos, etc. Subject, key ideas related to subject, emphasis where appropriate, conclusion, and a pleasant salutation are all you typically need.

Outline Format works well! It helps highlight ideas, it sets things up so people can see how ideas interrelate, and you can keep things brief and concise.

One key idea per e-mail, document, memo, plus sub-points is a good rule of thumb – more than that and you take the emphasis off what is important. If you have another key idea, send another terse document.

Instructions, e-mail (and wherever possible other documentation) – keep it short enough that it can be read at a glance – five-ten seconds. If you don't do this, it is very likely it will be 'tabled' until later and then often forgotten and discarded. If you need to add more material – attach it. Or present it in outline form in the e-mail body, and attach explanations, supporting evidence, etc.

> Follow-up instructions you give to a patient to see if they need clarification. It is often best to read the instructions out loud and then ask whether they have any questions. If there is any doubt, or to be doubly sure they understand, ask them to reiterate what they need to do.

Attachments: volume is not quality. Stick to clear, concise outlines with information presented in such a way that it can be understood quickly – again, preferably at a glance. Material should be directly relevant to key idea in e-mail/memo, nothing extra.

Documentation – ditto all the above, plus – Practice. You can save yourself (and others) a great deal of time if you learn to write in a clear, concise, descriptive manner with no added fluff.

Help others understand the need to keep business information professional, to the point, and as minimal as possible. [Other types of information sharing and more general e-mails should not get in the way of what needs to be focused on and accomplished professionally. It helps for people to be able to tell which is which at a glance.]

While keeping things terse is an important factor, make sure you are getting the key ideas across clearly.

Information flow

The truth is many things can get in the way of effective communication and information sharing: people's personalities, egos, forgetfulness, overwork, stress, resistant behavior, negativity, and so on. In the next few chapters we will discuss communication more specifically. You can develop and practice the skills and tools needed to effectively communicate in difficult situations.

Most importantly try to keep in mind that your fundamental purpose is patient care and the information flow throughout your workplace directly impacts everyone's ability to do your best for them.

Questions and Ideas for Contemplation

What are some roadblocks you feel might be getting in the way of information flow in your workplace? Make an effort to delineate these; then spend some time considering what you can do in your current position to help facilitate improving the overall network of information sharing at work.

Try to avoid blame, because that doesn't solve problems. There are always ways to make things better without negativity.

Be proactive in facilitating information sharing at work.

Chapter 12

Communicating Effectively with Difficult Patients

Much of what we have discussed already gives you important ideas, skills, and tools to mitigate problems with difficult patients. In this chapter we will discuss some specific ways you can use communications effectively to help you overcome difficulties as they arise.

A quick refresher

What you already can bring to the situation:

> When you maintain a calm, controlled, professional, caring approach you will have far fewer concerns right from the start.

> Opening up your communications right away with a patient can help immensely to calm their anxiety and concerns.

> Using your skills to understand and focus on a patient's needs, wants, and desires will further temper difficult concerns and can help redirect energy in positive ways.

> Showing through your work, your demeanor, and your communications that you are focusing on a patient's needs and concerns is a big step toward mitigating their negativity.

> Stay keenly aware of how you come across, what you say, and what you do. Through self-observation you acquire the ability to make positive action choices that will help you work through difficulties that arise.

> Facilitating information flow at work will help improve overall patient care.

Walking in the door

Good communications, especially with difficult individuals, start when you enter the room. Regardless of the behavior they are perpetrating upon you and probably others too, you need to remain professional and caring. Then you need to get them to focus on your intent – to help them. Once you achieve that, the vast majority of people, will give you the opportunity to do so.

Sometimes it is simply a matter of getting their attention and letting them know:

Get their attention – "Sir, sir,...sir...I am here to help you. Please let me know what I can do for you, right now, to help you with your concern."

Tell them your purpose – Offer to help with whatever it is that they are upset about.

> "Mrs. Smith, I can see you are very upset about something. Try to calm down and I will do everything I can to help you with your concern. I'm here to help."

It is a simple technique, but it works. People like to be catered to and to be the center of focus. Give them the opportunity for that and bingo – you have solved a ton of difficult people concerns!

Often it has to do with following up from this type of start by:

Helping them feel in control – Difficult people often just need to feel in control. When we allow them 'the floor' so to speak, they feel better and are more willing to go along with suggestions, ideas, tests, and so on that you need to accomplish. Help them stay in control by being willing to answer questions, offer explanations, give feedback, and so on.

Helping them feel safe – remember that fear factor! A little appropriate conversation at the right time about whatever you are currently trying to accomplish can make a world of difference.

Staying professional and calm – Critical point – Negativity breeds Negativity. At all costs, with any difficult person, you cannot show frustration, upset, defensiveness, etc. It can, and often does, set the stage for more difficulties. Stay within your professional, caring demeanor regardless of how 'jerky,' negative, or difficult they might be.

Being Positive – **always** – when you stay within your caring, professional persona, you create an atmosphere/aura that surrounds you. Over even a short period of time, it is tough for someone not to be affected by that. You don't have to be gushy or bubbly, but you do have to stay away from any form of negativity – even a frown can set a difficult person off on another tirade. You might be surprised at how little subtle 'positivities,' i.e. a smile, a light touch to the hand, a little kidding at the right moment, can change a curmudgeon into a softie. Try different things, such as....

Complimenting them/Thanking them/Appreciating them – for what they say and do that moves you and their treatment in the right direction. It is amazing what some simple things like a well-placed compliment or a 'thank you for telling me that', and so on, can do to a negative moment. Sometimes it seems like the last thing we want to do for someone who is giving us so much trouble is to offer them a compliment or thank them, but it is worth the effort, and it is surprising how effective it can be.

Remember: Positivity breeds Positivity!

Tell them, tell them, tell them

"Mr. Smith, this may be a bit uncomfortable, but I will help you through this procedure every step of the way. If you have any questions, please let me know. I want you to feel as comfortable and safe as possible."

"Miss Jones, I know you are worried about your test results. It is going to be a few more hours before we know anything, but I will stay on top of this and let you know as soon as something comes back. If you need anything at all, please ring your call button and one of the other Nurses or I will come as soon as possible. Please remember, though, that sometimes we are with other patients and it may take a moment or two."

People want to be kept informed. Whenever feasible, it is best to tell them. It is usually better to err on the side of too much information and detail, rather than too little, when it comes to a patient's needs and wishes.

Ask, ask, ask

"Is there anything else I can do for you right now?"

"I understand you are upset, Mr. Eldrige. What can I do to help?"

One of the most common problems in communicating is that we don't put into words what we are thinking. We know Mr. Eldrige is upset. When we say it out loud, we let him know that we know, which sets a completely different stage. We also can assume that he knows we are there to help, but when we actually 'say it,' it somehow becomes more real.

Communicating with really difficult patients

All of the above AND

Don't stop trying!

While their negativity, rudeness, resistance, etc., may be hard to take and especially difficult to put-up with while remaining calm and in control, it is the only thing that will work in the long haul.

Author's Note: This does work! From my professional experience as a counselor, mentor, and executive and personal coach for many years, I have had some very resistant clients and some who actually refused to talk with me – at first. What it took to get through to them was patience, positivity, and an openness on my part to accept them for who they were for the space and time they were with me. It always worked.

Violence or the threat of violence

Never put yourself or anyone else at risk. If a patient threatens you in any way physically, or is difficult to control, get help. Techniques discussed in this book can help, but they should never take precedence over your safety.

Harassment

You should not put up with any type of harassment from a patient. You have a right to stand up for yourself and to respond in a way that protects you and others. Often you can do this in a neutral or positive way, but you do need to be firm about these types of issues. (See Chapter 20 for specific information on dealing with Harassment concerns.)

Questions and Ideas for Contemplation

Working through specific scenarios you have encountered with difficult patients is an excellent way to start to envision putting these types of ideas and skills to work.

Questions? Scenarios?

Contact us at: responses2@difficultpeople.org.

Chapter 13

Solving Problems and Concerns

Patients expect you, and other medical/hospital personnel, to solve their problems and concerns. Whether it is something mundane, like getting them water or shifting their pillow, helping them to the bathroom, or something more involved, like helping ease their pain, assisting with a procedure, helping them through a medical crisis, and so on, is somewhat irrelevant – they want service. And it is not unusual for difficult patients to want it NOW!

Nurses are, in my opinion, the bulwark of the medical profession. You handle sophisticated equipment and tasks and yet, are also expected to do 'menial,' not-so-fun things, too (not sure emptying bedpans is at the top of anyone's list!). How you approach and handle this wide diversity of responsibilities will dictate your success with any given patient.

Approach, Focus, Communications

The skills and tools you use go back to these basics:

> Your over-all **approach** and demeanor as a caring professional

> Your **focus** on the patient and his/her needs, wants, and desires

> How effectively you **communicate** with them

Your success will be dependent on how the patient perceives your efforts on his/her behalf.

To make sure you are successful – talk, explain, ask.

The tough part

A demanding patient can be tough to deal with – especially if you have been on a long difficult shift, stress levels are high, and they just seem to want to add to the mix. That is why focus remains such an important tool. When you can zero in on a patient's concerns, they will be far more likely to move out of their demanding, rude, and negative behavior to accepting you for what you are trying to do for them.

One of the best ways to show focus is to ask them what they want, and then to follow that up with seeking more specificity if there is any question about their needs. Patients can help you solve their problems and concerns if you are open and willing to let them. It goes back to that 'control' issue. Give them the opportunity to have some control of their situation and it would be very rare for them not to back off from their negativity.

In the know

Patients often become upset and 'difficult' when they feel they don't understand what is happening to or with them. How much information are they receiving about their situation?

This goes to the idea of control – the more they know, in detail, about what is going on, their condition, what is about to transpire, what the results of some test are, etc. – the less likely to be worried and hence, demanding or difficult. AND the less likely they will continue to bother you and others.

Knowing gives a person a sense of control, and it definitely can relieve their stress.

> Author's Note: I had an old 'Country-type' Physician once who approached things fairly pragmatically. He was up to speed on all the latest knowledge, but he also stuck to some grass-roots notions. One of these was essentially, "If you can get above/on top of the pain; the patient will heal better." Frankly, from my own personal experience, I agree with him. However, what I want to emphasize here is not physical pain and the medicinal relief of pain, but psychological pain or distress.

'Not knowing' creates stress. Stress IS a form of pain – emotional pain. Stress can create worry, and hence more stress, and more pain, and so on. And as you know can lead to other physical concerns.

68

Solving concerns and problems for a patient can be as simple as keeping them informed and knowledgeable about anything and everything to do with their condition, which goes directly back to their needs, wants, and desires.

Yes, you want to address their presenting concern, e.g. "I have a migraine." But consider how much better your treatment would be received if you added to the medicine you gave them some sort of explanation, e.g...

> "One side effect of the procedure you just had can be a severe headache. I will give you medication the Doctor prescribed for this, however, it will help a great deal if you lie as quietly as possible and try to rest. Typically the pain will begin to dissipate after twelve hours." And so on.

> Even this brief effort on your part could help put a patient more at ease – more ease, less stress (for all concerned); less stress, faster healing. [Or so I believe and so did my old country Doc.]

Need to solve a patient's concern?

Be willing to:

Ask

Listen

Inform

Ask some more

Unfortunately the problem we often run into is we are overworked, stressed, and we don't always have the support we need to do our job to the best of our ability. That is why these few ideas become even more important. Focus on your patient(s) in the right way (positively!) and you will have fewer concerns to address in the long run and far fewer long-term problems with a difficult patient.

Questions and Ideas for Contemplation

As you can tell this Chapter is less about 'Problem Solving' than it is about how you can approach solving problems and concerns so that your professional success will not be hampered by patient distress. Most patients assume that their care-giver in any medical situation is competent, so what becomes important is how that care-giver goes about solving their problems and concerns, so that they feel cared for.

Be professional; but also focus on the humanity of the person you are dealing with.

Two good questions to ask yourself when you are dealing with any concern and especially when dealing with problems exacerbated by difficult behaviors are:

If I was this patient, and this was my concern, how would I want to be treated?

What would I want to know?

Chapter 14

Nurses as Liaisons, Mediators, Facilitators

"Mediation is the use of a neutral third party to help those in conflict find and agree upon an acceptable resolution by providing a process for reaching settlement."

(Orr, *American Journal of Bioethics*, Fall 2001, Vol. 1, #4)

Patients, Spouses, Significant Others, Relatives, Friends, Physicians, Coworkers, Supervisors – sometimes feel like you are stuck between a rock and a hard place? You probably know what it is like to be in a counseling situation with two belligerent people (or more)!

The scope of a Nurse's job is far-reaching, and it is not unusual for you to be caught in the middle of a difficult situation where good communication skills will be needed. Not that you should have to accept that role for any period of time, but it does happen, and it is better to be prepared, at least up until you can call in the cavalry – supervisor, Physician, psychologist, etc.

Liaison and Coordinator

Often it is an important part of your job to serve as a go-between from Physician to Patient/Patient to Physician; Patient to Coworker/ Coworker to...and so on. As in all communications where multiple parties are concerned, mistakes multiply the more 'go-betweening' there is. Coordinating things between parties have similar concerns.

To be at the top of your game

Always keep things clear, as simple as possible, short and to the point

Clarify

Important! Many mistakes are made when passing information along because there are slight misinterpretations of what has been said. One of the most critical skills you can develop is to seek clarification and specificity. This is key no matter what direction the information is flowing – as you know Physicians are not always clear about instructions either.

Seeking clarity requires a willingness to ask, as well as the ability to backtrack and paraphrase. The better you understand, the easier it will be to pass the information on correctly and understandably to the next person in the chain.

Repeat

Repetition almost never hurts' and almost always helps – and it helps **everyone** remember

A key tool is to ask the receiver to repeat back what you have said. This can be done directly, or you can be more subtle by asking them if they have any questions and asking them some questions about the information you have passed on. We can all be absent minded, especially if overworked and stressed. When something is important, it pays to make sure everyone gets it right.

Simplify

Sometimes the best way to pass on information is to put it in the most easily understood form possible while preserving the intent. This facilitates everyone's understanding and it can uncomplicate the transmission from point A to point B when you are receiving information. This can be accomplished by rephrasing back to the instigator the gist of the information – you will receive clarification, the information will be repeated, and you will make sure you got the information correct in the process – a winning situation all around.

When you are passing information on, be sure to keep things as clear and simple as possible. Fewer mistakes will be made and everyone will be happier in the long run.

Be Concise/To the Point

'Brevity is the Soul of Wit,' and it is smart when dealing with busy people. When it comes to remembering something and getting it right and when the information is needed and critical, it can make all the difference in the world.

Write it down

If there is any doubt about transmitting something clearly, or about making sure someone gets it right put it in writing. Plus, when it is in written form, it provides documentation if you need it.

Care in writing instructions so that they are clear, brief, but cover the ground needed for patient/spousal/relations understanding can be very effective in avoiding difficulties later. When in doubt as to whether someone understands – ask.

Your approach as a caring professional is also a key factor in all forms of communication at work, especially when coordinating ideas and events between people.

Mediator

While it would be nice to think that you wouldn't find yourself in a position where you have to serve as a mediator between parties, as you know it happens more often than not. Somehow you, the Nurse, the consummate professional caregiver, find yourself 'caught in the middle.'

In a sense, this should be a mark of pride for your profession. People expect you to be able to solve their problems, whether they are directly related to 'Nursing' or not. As a result, you get called upon to 'solve' concerns.

Important things to consider when serving as a Mediator

A calm, in control approach is the best. Keeping things on as even a keel as possible will help diffuse a difficult situation.

When you are forced into the position where you have to mediate a dispute, stay on top of key communication skills:

Gain everyone's attention; be the solid, in control force in the middle of the fray

Stay calm; your demeanor will help bring everyone back to center; use a calm, soothing, but firm and in control tone of voice

Offer to help, support, find answers, etc., "as much as feasible." It is important to say this as it has a calming effect. In other words, state specifically what you can and can't do.

Show concern and interest in helping and in being supportive. This can be all it takes to get everyone on the same page enough to work out whatever problems there are.

Open up communication: often (most often) upset, disputes, etc. are at the root caused by misunderstandings and poor communication. Getting people calm and talking can quickly dissipate concerns and open the door for better relations all the way around.

Get help if needed and feasible. Two neutral people can often have a much more calming effect than one.

Draw a line – you know what you are capable of handling. Don't try to do more than that, unless it is an emergency. Call in appropriate reinforcements as soon as feasible. You shouldn't have to provide extensive counseling services, etc.

Don't 'take sides.' Provide data, information, etc. that is accurate and appropriate to the issue at hand.

Encourage communication – use your communication skills to get people talking with each other. Try to move from 'being in the middle' to 'facilitating' as quickly as possible.

Facilitator

The real key to facilitating discussion or information flow is for you to be open and honest. In any conversation, the flow is set by all participants, but one person can make a great deal of difference by being willing to encourage others through their own ability to share openly and honestly. This can be further enhanced by:

Asking subtle and leading questions

Seeking clarity

Focusing on the other people present

Focusing on what is important to another person – being willing to ask them

Using non-verbal cues in an encouraging way – nods, eye contact, smiles, etc.

Allowing the other person time to respond – especially useful if they are shy and/or unresponsive

Following a lead or comment by encouraging someone to "go on"

Paraphrasing

Praising an idea

Thanking them for sharing– not necessarily just at the conclusion

Summarizing at the end of a conversation (or segment of conversation) – This shows you have been listening and paying attention. It is encouraging, supportive, and acknowledging and serves to recognize that what they have said is important. It also shows respect for their ideas, whether you agree with them or not.

Responsibilities

Your responsibility as a good communicator is not necessarily something you initially thought of when you chose Nursing as a profession. If you make the effort to continually improve your skills in working with others, learning what works and what doesn't, you will achieve a high level of professionalism that will make a major difference in your success at work.

Questions and Ideas for Contemplation

Your work as a liaison, mediator, and facilitator is a fertile field for personal growth. While it can be difficult at times to shoulder this 'extra' burden, it is one of the things that sets you and your profession apart. When you are willing to accept this challenge, you will take a step or two higher on the ladder of what humanity is all about.

People will appreciate your efforts.

Part IV

Succeeding with Difficult Patients

In this section of the book we will discuss in more detail Key Ideas centered around working with difficult situations and difficult people you may encounter in your work. All of the basic ideas, skills, and tools discussed up to this point serve as a foundation for your success. Now we will suggest ways to implement them toward more specific concerns.

Chapter 15

Difficult Patients: Key Ideas

Difficult Behaviors

It is often hard to separate a person from their way of presenting themself and when a person is 'in-your-face' it can be almost impossible. The truth is, however, that most people are not incorrigibly difficult. Even the very few who are, probably have some redeeming qualities, if we are willing to dig deep enough.

Key Ideas to Remember

Most difficult people don't see themselves as difficult. (Not even really difficult people!)

Most people who are being difficult to/with you, probably see you as being difficult as well. This can be a tough idea to accept, but it is often true.

They may be having a bad day, week, year, life. (We've all had a few bad days/weeks, we can afford to commiserate.)

They are undoubtedly frightened, and their current setting (hospital room, clinic room, procedure room, etc.) is most likely adding to their stress, upset, and nervousness.

When you can keep these ideas in the back of your mind it is easier to remain calm and in control and to **focus specifically on their behavior**, not on their 'difficultness' in general.

Where you focus is Key

By focusing on a specific behavior you have a better chance at being successful with someone than by focusing broadly on a perspective of them as a 'difficult person,' 'jerk,' etc.

Very important: your focus may be a key factor in their 'coming out of' their difficult behavior, BECAUSE difficult behavior is usually a cry for attention. Pay attention, really pay attention, to what a patient needs and wants ('Hey, it's me!' is often their inner scream) and you can begin to solve many issues right from the get-go.

For example:

> A demanding person – focus in on their demands, and how they are making those demands. You then have a chance of mitigating their difficult behavior as well as fulfilling their needs.

> A rude, obnoxious person – focus on what they are saying. How are they saying it? Does it give you any clues as to how to address their concerns? If not, what questions do you need to ask in order to find out? Or what do you need to say to move them out of this behavior and into more neutral or even positive territory?

> A resistant person – focus on what they are resistant to. How are they manifesting their resistance – silence, refusal to answer questions, refusal to move, etc? When you know this, you can help remove the obstacles creating their resistance, or know how to communicate with them better to ease their concerns.

IMPORTANT: there are always positive (best) and neutral (okay) ways to work with difficult behaviors and the people manifesting them. You get a wide variety of ideas in this text, but your best tools are the basics we have already discussed and your ability to adjust to differing situations presented. Keep in mind that all people are different – what may work with one person may not work in quite the same way with another. Be willing to change your approach as needed.

Find out

The sooner you can find out what a difficult patient's concerns are, the easier this all will be for you and them. By focusing on them, being willing to ask questions, and by listening carefully, you can often quickly move a person from their 'difficulty' into more open territory.

Couple this with your willingness to support, help, and care for their concerns and most often you will have solved presenting concerns. Important: you HAVE TO SAY IT:

> "Mr. Smith I am here to help you. I will do everything I can to support you through this difficult period."

> "Elsie, I know this is difficult for you. Let me help you and it will make it a lot easier for you."

> "Johnny, I know you are scared. Let's work together to get through this procedure. Can you tell me what you want me to do to help? Would you like me to hold your hand?"

> "Steve, I want to help. Can you tell me what is upsetting you?"

Again, talking can be very calming. If a patient is stressed, it can help a good bit to keep up an easy chatter that is supportive and caring.

Negativity

Negativity does tend to breed negativity. If you are dealing with a patient who seems to be pervasively negative, you have to be determined to be the opposite, because: positivity breeds positivity.

Author's Note: I have found that an easy-going, light, even humorous style can work well with negative personalities. I will banter away until I get a small smile, a bit of a positive reaction, and then I quickly move to encourage that...

> "What a pretty smile you have Beth, and I thought you were trying to keep it from me."

> "Now that's more like it. I knew there was someone special buried behind that frown..."

Just the effort on your part not to buy into their negativity can make a difference. By bringing positivity to the mix, it is hard for someone not to be affected.

If you are more 'business-like,' you can still learn to add some positivity:

> First and foremost, for both you and for them – relax. Being stiff or tense will only add to the stress of a difficult situation

> Add some positive chit-chat – what a nice day it is, compliments, how good the Doctor is they are going to see, how great the people are in the hospital, say 'Thank you' when they do something right or helpful, etc. There are always positive things you can say. The goal is to move them out of their current space, their negativity – you do that by 1) not buying into it and 2) creating something else.

Keep the ball rolling

Often a patient sees many people in the course of their medical treatment. While you may have success while you are with them, their fears and concerns can come flooding back as soon as the situation changes. Obviously there are many situations where you can't control who else, or what else, impacts a patient. However, you can still help the continuing process of keeping them on a more even keel by 'spreading the word.'

Tell your coworkers, the Physician(s), etc. what you have done and what has worked. No one likes to deal with difficulty, and most everyone will appreciate the heads up.

When you have a second: pop your head in the room and say 'hi,' 'bye' (if your shift is ending), 'how're things going?' and so on. Remember to smile! It takes only a few seconds and this can really make a difference to a patient. It feels good to have someone remember you; to feel that someone cares.

In general, keeping things positive and light-hearted throughout your workplace on a daily basis helps everyone.

Grumpy, Grumpy, Discontent

Some people do seem intent on not enjoying life – be patient and stick to your positivity guns. Positivity CAN work in the most difficult of circumstances if someone is willing to keep up the effort.

Tired, Sick, Over-worked?

When we are under the gun or the weather, these are tough times to deal with difficulties in others, but you still have to find that positivity if you want to stay on top of things. If at all possible, take a few moments to rejuvenate. Even five minutes with your eyes closed, completely relaxed can recharge your energy and positivity for another few hours. [See Chapter 25, "Taking Care of Yourself" for more ideas related to this.]

When in doubt

Get back to the basics – who you are as a caring professional and the multitude of skills you bring to the table.

Alcohol and Drugs

As medical professionals you must deal with all types of personalities and behaviors. Behaviors that are exacerbated by drugs and/or alcohol can cause critical concerns to you at work.

Please keep the following key ideas in mind:

> Never put yourself or anyone else at risk. If you feel you need assistance, get it. It's better to be safe!

> By all means stay calm, professional, and caring. All of the

skills and techniques discussed in this book, can be helpful, but keep in mind that substance-affected behavior may not follow 'logical' patterns. Be prepared for anything.

If you deal regularly with this type of concern, maintain your own self-worth, health, and personal feelings. Your stress and upset can and will affect others. Take care of you!

Be firm, in control, and let the patient know very clearly what you can and can't do. Patient's who are demanding medication will not likely listen to reason. Get back-up help if you need to.

Know the guidelines established by your place of work for serious patient concerns. They may be what you need to fall back on if the situation escalates and threatens to get out of control.

Be kind, positive, and understanding whenever you can.

Remember:

Your professionalism sets the stage for controlling the situation.

Your ability to show understanding and caring can often help mitigate many concerns.

Good, positive communication is critical

Keep them informed

Be willing to ask and to listen to them regardless of their condition. The act of listening uncritically and supportively may be what they need to feel cared for.

Let them know (Tell them!) you are there for them (even if you can't give them the drugs they want). Your caring support may make all the difference in the world.

Questions and Ideas for Contemplation

What you focus on really can make a major difference in your success with/in difficult situations. Try separating the difficulty (the behavior) from the actual person. A good exercise is to do this for a week and jot down your observations. You can do this at work and in your every day life. Take particular note of how this exercise changes your perceptions. You will find that you feel more in control in any difficult situation.

Chapter 16

Dealing with Aggressive Patients

Aggressive personalities

Aggression can take many forms: a person can be rude and obnoxious, belligerent, bossy or bullying, explosive, and so on. Your most important skill is to NOT react to whatever their presenting behavior is.

IMPORTANT: Your safety and the safety of others is paramount. Never put yourself or anyone else at risk. If you feel you need help, get it.

Gain their attention

Whether a person is shouting, being rude, obnoxious, or bullying, your first key step is to let them know you are there to help:

> Repeat their name or say 'Sir,' or 'Ma'am' over and over again, until they stop ranting

> Maintain eye contact

> A light touch on a shoulder or arm may help, but be judicious with this. See how the situation unfolds. Ask, if it is okay to hug them, or touch them – for instance, on the shoulder, arm, or hand.

Your second step is to let them know:

> That you are willing and able to help

> That you want to understand their concerns

> That you will do everything in your power to support them and to help ease their concerns

Remember it is key to actually state these things – more than once, if necessary

If the presenting behavior continues, or they lapse back into negativity, you may have to start over. You can also make a difference by saying something about what you appreciate, or what you need to do your job better:

> "Mr. Johnston it will be most helpful for me to assist you if you can try to remain calm. I am here to help you in any way I can and it is easier if I can understand your needs, so I can address them."

> "Thanks for calming down. I want you to know I am here for you. What can I do for you right now to ease your concerns?"

> "I sincerely appreciate your support and respect, Mrs. Smith. It makes my work so much better."

Important point: you can say these things even if there is very little improvement. Suggesting the type of behavior you like to see can help and can open a difficult person's eyes to their own negativity if done in positive and subtle ways. These types of 'sideways' hints can and will help. And they are so much better than something less positive. Also – make sure you are sincere. Any hint of sarcasm or negativity can make things worse. The more positive you are and the less affected by their negativity, the better.

For example, here are some ways NOT to say things:

> "Mr. Johnston I can't do my job well if you keep yelling at me."

> "I'm sorry, Mrs. Smith, but I don't have to put up with your negativity. Please treat me with respect."

> "I think that's about enough of your shouting. I'm a professional and expect to be treated courteously."

These statements are valid and you have every right to think them, but verbalizing them is not going to make the patient feel any better, nor are they likely to effectively change their behavior toward you.

> "You always have a choice between
> being right and being kind...choose being kind."
>
> (Wayne Dyer)

There are always more positive ways to say things. Practice this technique and you will have far fewer difficulties with patients.

Here's a way to address even a very upset patient, positively –

> "Bob, I can tell you are very angry about something. Please tell me what it is, so I can address it. I can't help unless I know what you are upset about. I am here to help you."

Ease their worry, their pain, their fear, their stress

Simple, relatively basic and easy to do IF we remember that these are what most often drive difficult behaviors.

Also important: don't forget to keep the positive banter up once you get a word in edgewise. Whether you are asking them questions, working through a procedure, maintaining your focus on their concerns, keeping them focused in a more positive direction, and so on, these all can help to keep them out of negativity. Remember to keep the focus on them – people, especially difficult people, like to be appreciated, to be the center of attention, and to feel 'in control.'

In control

Feeling in control is one of the foremost motivations of aggressive (and even passive-aggressive) personalities. Most of the time you can allow them to have that sense of control, without giving up anything yourself.

Think about the difficult behavior they are manifesting:

> Are they being rude or abrasive?

> Insulting?

> Yelling, angry, upset?

> Pushy, bossy, bullying?

These all scream "Me, Me, Me" and "Mine, Mine, Mine"

> Pay attention to the "Me" – go ahead, focus on them and their needs

> Bingo – most of the time, problem solved

These types of behaviors also say 'I'm afraid,' 'I need to get on top of being afraid and I can do that by hiding it with these behaviors and these other emotions,' 'This is how I deal with my fear, by trying to control others and the situation.'

Give them control by addressing their concerns, their needs, and by paying supportive attention to them.

Hint: There are many suggestions in this book for 'paying attention' in positive ways, but you know yourself the best, and you can develop a repertoire of skills and strategies as you try different things out.

Being alone

Think about this: patients often spend a fair amount of time (sometimes a lot of time) alone in their room (whether a clinic setting or hospital or even home care). That is time where their concerns and worries can become exacerbated. Your kindness can make a major difference to them in a short period of time.

> Author's Note: I can remember a situation when I was in the Walter Reed Medical Center many years ago with a type of blood concern that had the Doctors perplexed. A Nurse had asked me to strip down to my briefs and I ended up sitting on the end of a metal hospital gurney with no cover on it or sheet, in not much more than my birthday suit for a long half hour by myself. It was pretty cold, so I was just short of putting my clothes back on when a Physician entered, did a cursory exam, and then opened the door and shouted, "Come in here, Come in here, you have got to see this!"

> Well, needless to say, I thought I was about to die. He followed that statement up, as several Nurses and Doctors flooded into the room, with, "Isn't this the worse case of Acrocyanosis you've ever seen?"

> Then, of course, I knew I was a goner. Figured I had only moments to live.

> I didn't find out until that evening, when I talked with my brother, that I had the 'dread' disease of 'poor circulation

in the extremities." Heck, I could have told them that – my fingers and toes always get cold in the winter.

Just goes to show you what sitting alone in a room in an uncomfortable situation can do for you, not to mention the lack of consideration and lack of information I was being given. Lucky for them I wasn't a difficult person!

Things NOT to do

Make the effort to look at everything as much as possible from a CAN DO perspective, but here are some actions/reactions to avoid:

Never:

> Shout back
>
> Show anger, frustration, upset
>
> Get defensive (watch your reactions, facial expressions, gestures, physical actions, etc.)
>
> Complain to them, blame them, etc. (Remember – negativity breeds negativity)
>
> Show any negativity
>
> (Or leave someone sitting on a metal gurney for a half hour in their skivvies!)

As soon as you do, you will have erased all the positive work you have done to that point.

Yes, there are really difficult, curmudgeonly people out there, however, your actions and reactions must stay within your caring professional approach – always.

If you need a break from difficulty, find a way to take it. It is far better than showing your upset to a patient.

Important Idea

Really difficult people, especially aggressive people, **EXPECT us to react to their negativity.** When we don't, it takes the air out of their balloon. When we react and act from a solid base of

89

kindness, we throw them off their 'preferred' method of dealing with others and they will, in a sense, be forced to act differently.

**If we react negatively to their difficult behavior,
we are reinforcing that behavior.**

It is worth keeping this idea in your mind when you are knee-deep in a situation with an aggressive personality.

Questions and Ideas for Contemplation

It is easy to be intimidated and affected by an aggressive person. When we can take a step back and say to ourselves, 'I don't need to buy into this behavior,' it gives us that instant to refocus ourselves so we can maintain our calm, in control, professional self.

The best way to accomplish this is through practice. Initially, try mentally rehearsing scenarios with difficult aggressive patients. Visualize how you would normally react to their negativity; then, envision how things would be different if you maintain your composure and simply go about your positive, supportive caring of this patient.

Then try it in real life. Be sure to self-observe and adjust to the situation as you need to. Soon you will develop more and more self-confidence and control.

Chapter 17

Dealing with Passive-Aggressive/ Resistant Patients

Some patients respond to stress and fear by resisting your efforts to help. Passive-aggressive personalities are not 'in-your-face' difficult, but they can be equally exasperating because it is hard to get through their ability to stonewall every attempt you make to assist them.

They may manifest their upset in a variety of ways:

Not talking – won't answer questions, won't respond, refuse to engage

Physically resist what you need to do – a patient won't turn over if asked, won't raise an arm, won't put on their gown, etc.

Display resistance at any suggestion, offer to help, and so on – they sit with arms and legs crossed at end of a hospital bed; refuse to get up and go to the bathroom following an operation; etc.

What can you do?

Keep in mind the fear factor – resistance is a form of protection. Understand that they are simply trying to protect themselves and maintain control of the situation in the only way they feel they can for this moment in time. Thus, your best offense is to help them to feel safe and in control.

Talk (even if they won't)

Open up communications regardless of whether or not they respond or not to your efforts. The more you offer, the more likely they will be to soften up a bit and feel comfortable. When they do, say something to encourage them further by being complimentary – help them and make sure you listen carefully to what they say, etc.

Things you can say that will help

Offer explanations about everything you can – what you need to do, who you are, what is important to them, why you need to have them do something, and so on. The more open you are with them, the more likely they will begin to relax. The more they know, the more in control they will feel. It may be obvious to you, but it is not necessarily obvious to them. It is likely they are resisting because not only is it not obvious to them, they are probably frightened. Explain in detail, if necessary, as both your continuous effort and your openness may eventually have an effect.

Be understanding; be willing to say what you recognize and understand:

> "Beth, I know you are frightened. Let's see if we can find a way to make this better for you. I want you to tell me what works for you and what doesn't. If something bothers you, let me know. We will try to get through this together...."

Keep up the chatter. However, always stay on top of things by observing carefully how they respond. With a reticent patient you may want to pause for long moments to see if they want to say something. Start by asking simple questions that require easy answers. They may answer with a nod or shake of the head to begin with, but that's progress – encourage them from there. [This is also important with Passive patients.]

Be honest about everything you can: openness about what you need to do, what they need to do, what is going to transpire when the Doctor comes in, etc. Knowing helps dissipate their fears. If they ask a question, be as forthright as possible when answering and be sure to follow through with something akin to, "What else can I help you understand." In other words, once the door has opened a crack, get your foot in the door and open it wider.

Use words like: 'I understand,' or 'I'm trying to understand,' and 'I care,' 'I'm trying to help,' 'I'm here for you,' 'What you feel is important,' and so on.

Encourage, support, and compliment them – especially if they respond in any way toward what you are trying to do. Thank them for even small successes, and so on. Keep talking and keep up the positivity:

> "See that wasn't so difficult. Now, let's see if we can move the other arm. Good, you are doing great, John. I know it is hard and you are very sore, but it is important for you to move or you'll just stiffen up more. Great, that's perfect. Now let's try your left..."

Sometimes it really helps to have Nurses offering a kind of Grandmotherly (or Grandfatherly) support. You may want to think of this imagery for a moment and see how it feels for you. [People want to feel safe and there is nothing safer, in my mind, than remembering my Italian grandmother's hugs and smiles.] At any rate, keep in mind that their need to be safe is a major issue with passive-aggressive, resistant patients. (As well as with Passive patients, see next Chapter.)

Be patient

It may take some time for a person to come around. However, it will invariably happen if you are patient, stay positive, and keep at it. Work with your coworkers and other care-givers on this as well. Unless they understand what you are doing and why, they may try other approaches that will result in more resistance.

> Author's Note: I have worked with very resistant clients who came to sessions and simply sat angrily in a chair opposite me. I talked, I sat, I stayed calm, I maintained my friendly professionalism – they eventually opened up, and ultimately we developed a positive working relationship as I continued to encourage them.

Must do's

Sometimes there are things you have to do that are important for the patient for treatment to be successful and there isn't much wiggle room time-wise – the key here is to talk them through it even if they continue to resist. Your calm, caring professionalism will help and you can set the stage for them eventually relaxing their resistance by doing whatever needs to be done.

An example

You have a patient that needs to get up and move or they will have serious side-effects from their surgery. Unfortunately, in spite of everyone's efforts, they refuse to budge from their bed. Help them through the preliminary stages and talk with them all the way through your efforts:

> About why it is important for them

> About how you understand that it is uncomfortable and difficult for them

> About exactly what you are doing and why (i.e. moving their arm, etc.)

> And so on. Keep it up throughout.

Most often, they will begin to relax if you approach it this way. Be kind, as gentle as possible, and do it in short sessions, if feasible. Offer encouragement, support, compliments, and say thank you throughout the process.

Your demeanor is KEY!

Remember positivity breeds positivity. Yes, it may take time, but your kindness and caring will make a difference with resistant patients.

Also keep in mind that gentle appropriate touching can be very healing. You can quickly tell if a patient is uncomfortable with anything you do. A good rule of thumb is to ask them or to state it: [I always ask my clients the first time, i.e. if they like hugs; and I always tell them or ask them if I am going to touch them, i.e. their shoulder, reach out to hold their hand, etc.]

Other forms of positive physical expression can be more automatic: high fives; pats on the back, or the latest – touching knuckles [I know, it's kind of a 'guy thing.']

Questions and Ideas for Contemplation

Resistant patients can seem more difficult to deal with than aggressive, in-your-face, patients. Your keys to success are in creating an atmosphere that is safe for them. Try imagining a scenario where you walk into a clinic room and the patient is sitting on the edge of a chair, arms folded protectively across their chest, legs crossed, a scowl on their face – what's next?

Observe what you say and do that helps ease their worries. Can you create a positive, receptive patient, from someone who obviously isn't going to be cooperative from the get-go?

Chapter 18

Dealing with Passive Patients

A classic passive patient would essentially not respond to you –
what you say, what you do, and so on. It is not because they are
being resistant to your overtures or ministrations – they may have
given up caring, be so frightened that they have withdrawn into
themselves, or are extremely uncomfortable and don't know how
to respond safely.

Safety first

As with passive-aggressive personalities, safety is an important
issue. Create a positive, safe, open environment and typically they
will begin to come out of their shells. Use many of the positive
techniques described in the previous chapter, especially:

    Supportive, caring, open communications

    Safe and appropriate touching may work wonders

    Compliments, encouragement, appreciation

Asking

Unresponsive patients may not answer questions, but it doesn't
hurt to ask because –

    It shows you are focusing on them

    It acknowledges who they are and that they are important

    It shows respect

    It encourages them to open up

Be patient

Whenever possible, be patient with passive personalities. They
may take a good bit of caring, kindness, and gentle cajoling to

come around. That first hint of a smile or a glimmer in their eyes will tell you that you are making a difference.

Assisting them kindly and gently will also help. Keep up positive communications by describing what you need to do, what you are doing, why, and so on. Your tone of voice, kindness, support, encouragement, and gentleness can make all the difference toward getting them to come around.

All that fear

Have you ever thought about the myriad of reasons a patient might be 'deathly' afraid of the situation they are facing?

> Fear of needles
>
> Fear of sterile surroundings (associated with previous pain, discomfort)
>
> Fear of Doctors (previous experience)
>
> Fear of the unknown (very common)
>
> Fear of not being in control of their life and future
>
> Fear of pain in general

All of these and many more are possible. Talking about and through fears, what is happening, what is about to happen, how they feel, how they might feel as the result of procedure or test, what concerns them, etc., whether you get a response or not, can begin to help ease their unease.

Beyond Hope

If you occasionally, or even regularly, work with patients who have chronic and/or terminal illnesses, encouragement may seem like a broken record not worth playing. The truth is, people will eventually respond to kindness and whatever hope there is to be found. Offer them whatever you can. Case in point:

> Author's Note: I once wrote a note to my elderly, failing mother. For a long time she had been complaining quite demonstratively about this and that and how she didn't feel useful anymore. She wondered aloud to whoever

98

would listen, 'Why am I still here?' 'Why don't I just die?' 'Why is God keeping me here?'

In that letter, the gist of what I said was, 'Maybe as our life runs down, our purpose here on earth is simply to be nice to all those people who we come in contact with   to share whatever kindnesses we can; to be positive for them in spite of our own pain and suffering, to offer whatever wisdom we might from our own experiences.'

She had that letter read to her every day for the last six months of her life.

Maybe we can't solve their problems or heal their illnesses, but there are always ways we can help their lives be just a little bit better. Perhaps, we can still show them how precious life is even when it seems to be going against them.

When we make the effort, we can make a difference in people's lives, and you, as Nurses, have that opportunity every day. It is not just about providing a service, providing treatments and medicines, taking tests and making diagnoses, or doing procedures – it is very much about treating people with dignity and humanity and loving kindness.

Questions and Ideas for Contemplation

One good perspective to have with passive/resistant patients (and also passive-aggressive personalities) is to try to imagine yourself in their shoes. This type of understanding/empathy can help you make positive decisions in how you approach them and how you approach treatments and procedures. You can never entirely know what a patient is bringing to the table, but it is definitely worth trying to understand things from their perspective.

Chapter 19

Really Difficult Patients

Some people really do seem to be, well, jerks. Whatever it is that has happened in their lives to bring them to the point where they are, they just can't seem to deal with others without causing disruption and perturbation. When I think of a 'really difficult person' I think of someone who causes concerns with many/most of the people they interact with. While they may not realize the havoc they are causing, it is tacitly (and sometimes not so quietly) agreed that they are pervasively disruptive to a team or group.

So that raises the questions – can you be successful with really difficult people and their over-the-top behaviors? And if so, how?

First

Take care of yourself and those around you. Any potentially dangerous person or situation should be dealt with accordingly – get help. You should never put yourself or anyone else at risk.

Positivity breeds Positivity

In the face of pervasive negativity you sometimes wonder if anything can help – the truth is, if you stick to your guns (remember that calm, in control, caring professional you are) you can succeed.

> Author's Note: I have met the opposite of the extreme negative personality several times in my life and hands down they trump any negativity they encounter – they are infectiously positive. Even the worst grump cannot help but roll over and smile when they are in the room.

You may not be an outgoing, always smiling, bubbly-type person. You probably see yourself somewhere in the neighborhood of, likeable, kind, always trying to be positive, supportive, and professional – that's enough, IF –

You stick to your guns!

and don't let their negativity and disruptive behavior change who you are and how you present yourself.

A really difficult person is often out to yank your chain. They want and expect you to: cower, defend yourself, fight back, get angry, get upset, feel guilty and ashamed, and so on.

Key Idea

When they don't get what they expect, you have changed their world a bit – or a lot.

Stick to it long enough, and even the densest of people will get the idea that you can't 'be bought,' i.e. that you won't buy into their negativity.

When you don't buy into their negativity, they are essentially forced to change their behavior because they are not getting what they want – which is, fundamentally, to control you and the situation.

As detailed in previous Chapters, control is a major issue. Give them control by focusing on them and supporting them through their concerns, offering to listen to them, to help, and so on. Don't give them the type of control they want by reacting to their negativity. Even the most disagreeable person's difficult behavior will abate if it 'isn't working,' because it isn't 'fun' anymore. It is not getting them the results they want. That is when you want to fill the gap with more positive things by:

Paying them positive attention

Asking them what they need, want, and desire

Listening carefully to their concerns (even their complaints, blame, etc. – just stay professional and calm)

Drawing them out more and more, and keeping them occupied with your positive chatter

Keeping them informed – another way to offer them 'control' or the sense of being in control

Maneuvering them out of their negativity should they return to it.

Treating them respectfully and kindly, regardless of their presenting negative behaviors

Expect to be treated respectfully and professionally

You always have this right. Make sure if you use the type of statement below that you say it calmly with no hint of negativity in your voice, gestures, or facial expressions. Be polite, even if they haven't been. Observe yourself so you don't sound defensive.

> "Mr. Jones, I am here to do everything I can in my power to help you. I will treat you the best way I know how. I would sincerely appreciate it if you would be willing to treat me with kindness and respect, too."

Humor

Humor can be quite effective in very difficult situations, if you feel confident about it and have a good handle on what you are doing and what to expect. Sometimes a bit of humor will be just the right thing to take the edge off of a negative encounter.

To a belligerent, complaining, blaming patient – go ahead and put on an act:

> "Mrs. Smith, well I never! Are you trying to get to me or something? Do you do that to all your Nurses, or am I special? Come on you can do better than that."

Again, you have to be confident, know your stuff, and feel pretty self-assured that you can handle whatever comes next. The result can be anywhere from:

> Confusion, i.e. you have stopped them in their tracks, and they don't know what to make of your antics. This gives you an opening to continue bantering with them, trying to get them further out of their space and into some more neutral, or positive, ground.

They laugh and realize they have been a bit of a pain in the butt and as a result you have already worked wonders with them.

They look at you like you are crazy and launch into another tirade.

Reactions to humor are not always predictable, but then, neither are really difficult people. Be careful and intelligent about how you use humor, and back off from it quickly if it doesn't seem to be helping.

The Art of Apologizing

Another way to put the ball into a difficult person's court, i.e., to let them have more of a sense of control, is to apologize. There are many ways to do this without accepting guilt:

"I'm sorry you are so angry, Mr. Johnston. Can I help?"

"I'm really sorry you feel you haven't been treated well here. Tell me what I need to do to help make this experience better for you?"

This type of 'apology' doesn't hurt you, or anyone else, and it very well may assuage a patient enough to allow you to move into a better relationship with them.

Plus! It is important to apologize if you have made a mistake, even if it really isn't 'your fault.'

"I'm very sorry I could not get here quickly Mrs. Smith, we had an emergency with one of the other patients. You know I want you to be comfortable, and I will come as soon as I can to help."

If it is a small error or oversight on your part, or someone else's, then it is plain good business to apologize sincerely, ensure the patient that you will always do your best, and move on. In these cases avoid offering excuses or pointing your finger away from yourself.

Getting help

Another wise practice to embrace, if everything you are doing just doesn't seem to be helping, is to ask someone else to join you. It can be very effective to have a second person working the same magic with a very difficult person.

It is fairly typical for a negative individual to feel powerful and in control when they can 'beat-up' on one person, but throw two calm and in-control people in their path and they start to lose those feelings of superiority. It doesn't always work, but it is a good tactic to consider.

Important to note: The purpose isn't to 'gang up' on a patient, but to have support if and when you need it. Both of you need to stay calm, caring, professional, and to continue to use the positive skills and techniques you have learned in this book.

This two-person approach is also helpful because you can increase the positive banter and attention you give a particular patient. Keep in mind that positive attention can work wonders, and difficult patients often respond when they feel they are being paid attention to. It may take up more time than you and other Nurses may wish to give, but it may be well worth it if it helps keep this person under control and keeps them from spreading their havoc throughout your facility.

Out-of-Control Patients

You will sometimes encounter patients who have lost control psychologically, mentally, physically. Loss of control may be caused by many factors including alcohol, drugs, hysteria, fear, etc.

While many of the ideas and skills discussed in this book may help you when you are dealing with an out-of-control patient/situation it is important to get help. Many work places have recommendations, guidelines, and procedures for handling these types of situations. Please familiarize yourself with them.

Another important way to address these types of concerns is to raise the issue in appropriate meetings where this can be discussed openly with the entire staff.

Safety is paramount: yours, the rest of the staff, and all the patients.

Don't forget

Communication throughout your place of business, and especially with team members who will be in contact with or affected by this patient, are critical. Make an effort to keep the information flowing from person to person. Help others understand what you are doing, what you have tried with this patient, what seems to work, and pass on recommendations to the next person in line. Everyone will appreciate your efforts – Physicians, coworkers, supervisors, and staff.

Also, keep in mind that your success with this patient today, may mean that the next time they are in, or the next shift you have with them, will most likely be considerably easier.

Keys for you

Be patient. Get support. Take time for yourself when dealing with a difficult patient. Pat yourself on the back for the positive things that you accomplish. Treat yourself for your good work.

Taking care of you is good for everyone.

Questions and Ideas for Contemplation

Everyone has a horror story about certain types of patients. Write yours down with as much detail as you can remember and share with colleagues in an open discussion or at a seminar. Discuss different successes, strategies, options, etc.

Want to get our opinion about a difficult patient concern or situation? E-mail us at responses2@difficultpeople.org. We enjoy hearing from you and will make every effort to respond to your query. Please be patient as our response will be dependent upon the number of queries we receive.

Chapter 20

Sexual/Physical Harassment

You should never tolerate behaviors that are inappropriate.

Note: many companies address these issues in their employee handbooks. Use these types of documents as a reference point for further understanding and action. Regulations may dictate how you should respond to inappropriate behavior/actions by anyone. It is important to read these documents thoroughly and to take appropriate action as recommended in them. Ultimately, how you approach these concerns will be your decision.

> Author's Note: I have written about Sexual Harassment in detail in some of my other works: see *Succeeding with Difficult Bosses*, and *Succeeding with Difficult Coworkers*, for an in-depth look at these specific relationships in the work place. Some of the material below is excerpted from these books.

Sexual Harassment

Essentially the legal description for sexually inappropriate behavior is whether *a reasonable* woman or man would find the behavior to be sexual harassment. Obviously this leaves some questions about exactly how this might be interpreted by our legal system.

However, what is most important is how the behavior affects you. If YOU feel that a behavior is inappropriate or offensive, it is probably worth taking initial steps to curtail it/deal with it by bringing your concerns forward to an authority figure, appropriate department at work, and/or to the person(s) perpetrating the behavior.

Discrimination

Discrimination is treating someone differently because of some characteristic or trait.

For example:

Race or ethnicity

Creed or religion

On the basis of gender

Handicapped individuals

Specific laws cover these issues and appropriate authorities, human resources departments, and government sources can provide current information. NOTE: If at some point you feel the need to pursue your concern legally, please contact an appropriate agency and/or get a lawyer qualified in this area.

Prejudicial behavior

Prejudices can be very concerning but unfortunately they are often legally, ethically, and practically very hard to define and pin down. Well-documented concerns, however, can and should be addressed if they are causing significant problems and discomfort at work. It is not unusual for people to have minor, or even major prejudices of which they are unaware. Drawing attention to your concern with the perpetrator may be all that is necessary for the behavior to cease.

Dealing with inappropriate, harassing, discriminatory, and prejudicial behaviors from patients

Dealing with these issues in a care/service environment can be particularly difficult. However – and this is important – **if you are uncomfortable**, you should do something to alleviate your concerns. How you deal with them is based on several factors:

Workplace guidelines (important to know)

Legal issues (when in doubt, find out; this is typically the bailiwick of Human Resources, but your business may also have a legal department)

How YOU feel you should handle it

You should weigh each of these factors carefully.

Author's Note: With my wide range of experiences from administrator to counselor and coach I have had to deal with harassment and discriminatory issues from many perspectives. I have seen people who wished to deal with the issue themselves, and did so quite successfully. I have assisted others both as a mentor and as a mediator, and I have overseen pursuing these concerns in different ways.

Always seek help if you feel the need. Legal and supportive help are often available at work. Supervisors should be able to offer guidance. Most importantly you should not 'let it slide' as putting up with these types of behaviors, particularly over the long haul, can be very demeaning and devastating. You have the right and should make an effort to do something to alleviate the concern.

Nurses

As caring professionals, Nurses learn to deal with a wide range of difficulties throughout their workday and workweek. In many ways I believe you develop an inner personal strength that gives you the self-confidence to deal with many issues from a position of personal power. Sometimes all it takes with a patient (person) who is harassing you is a kind comment that indicates to them that you feel the behavior is inappropriate. You have every right to do this:

> "Mr. Smith, I want you to know that I find some of the comments you make and your sexual innuendos to be highly inappropriate. I would appreciate it if you would refrain from these types of statements in the future."

Simple, direct, to the point – the vast majority of people will understand that this is a wake up call and will stop doing what they are doing immediately. If it will help you feel more comfortable, it may be appropriate to make this type of statement with a supervisor present.

Another example:

> "Miss Jones, I need to tell you that I feel very uncomfortable when you make disparaging comments about others. I believe in treating everyone, regardless of their ethnic or cultural heritage, with kindness and respect. I trust you feel the same way."

It is important to say what you mean in a calm, clear voice that cannot be misunderstood. Try to remain neutral and non-defensive. Try to phrase what you need to say as kindly as possible, without being strongly accusatory. Always phrase your comments in the form of taking responsibility for your feelings. In other words avoid saying, "You make me..." Instead, say, "I feel that..." Another good idea is to work out what you want to say ahead of time and then write it down and keep it if you ever need to support what you have said/done. Otherwise be sure to write it down immediately after you have said it.

Often people really do not understand how they come across to others and will be very embarrassed about the whole situation. [Author's Note: Every time I have assisted in these types of situations the behavior has been curtailed immediately and no further concerns ever arose.]

Important: Always document any incidences that make you truly uncomfortable. Be sure to be very specific about details – what was said by the perpetrator, what you said and how you responded, dates, and so on. Documentation may be very important if you need to take further steps.

Choices

Discussing your concerns with a trusted person helps you document the whole process and can provide you with tremendous support. DO NOT keep these types of concerns to yourself. It is very important to let someone else know what you are concerned about and why. Be willing to be open and specific even if the whole situation is embarrassing and awkward at first.

If anyone has been witness to any of these incidents, ask them if they would be willing to witness your account. Whether they do or not, note their presence.

If there is another person at work who shares these same concerns, talk to them about what you are doing and ask them if they would like to keep their own records and/or work with you on resolving this joint issue. You can document your conversation with them whether they are willing to help back you up or not.

If you do not feel comfortable handling this by yourself, be sure you seek appropriate assistance for your situation and place of work – supervisor, mentor, Human Resources, or all-of-the-above.

Real jerks

There are some people who, for whatever reasons, don't seem to understand the whole concept of humanity and appropriateness. You don't have to put up with any form of harassing behavior and you should do something about it:

> Report to appropriate person/agency at work

> Follow through if the concern continues; make sure that everyone takes this seriously

> Get legal help/advisement if you feel the need and support

> Keep detailed documentation of everything that has happened and everything you have done

Very important

Your safety and well-being, as well as the safety and well-being of all those who work with you, is of paramount importance. When in doubt, take the actions that are best for you and others.

Questions and Ideas for Contemplation

Be sure to take care of yourself during any time you are dealing with unethical, inappropriate behavior. It can be a very stressful time. Support and understanding from friends and relatives is particularly helpful. I believe that sharing your concerns with a trusted relative or friend is essential throughout this whole process. This is a very heavy burden to carry alone.

Discussing this issue with colleagues and supervisors, ahead of any actual concerns, is an excellent way of knowing what your choices are at your place of work. Talking through experiences with your colleagues can also be very valuable. Share your successes and techniques – this helps everyone grow.

Part V

Other Issues

In this section of the book we will consider briefly some of the other critical relationships you have in your work-life, as these can indirectly have a marked impact on your work with patients. The knowledge, skills, and tools you have been introduced to throughout this text can serve as a foundation for working with others.

Chapter 21

Dealing with Difficult Families and Loved Ones

Stress

It is quite common for family members and loved ones to be as affected, and sometimes even more upset, than a patient in your care. As a Nurse you can find yourself in a position in which you are dealing with several concerns related to a single case. Your most important skill in dealing with these types of situations is maintaining your calm, professional approach and keeping communication lines open.

Information is often Key

People want to understand and know:

What is happening

What is about to happen

What the diagnosis is

What the prognosis is

What you are going to do about it (whether you can or not, and often whether it is your responsibility or not)

What you are going to do in the future

Who, What, Where, Why, How much, etc., etc....

Provide the information and assurances you can to the families and loved ones. As with patients, good, open, honest communications are best.

When there are proprietary concerns your best tool is to be honest about what it is you can and can't say to them:

> "Mr. And Mrs. Smith, I know you are concerned about your son, but I am not at liberty to discuss this with you. Dr. Johnston is the attending and responsible Physician and he will let you know everything he can as soon as he can."

It is far better to be honest about what you can and can't say, than to beat around the bush.

Important: These types of proprietary issues are common in the medical field. Be sure you have a good understanding founded in discussions with Physicians, Supervisors, Human Resources, and other appropriate sources at work, so you know precisely what the guidelines are ahead of time. When in doubt about a specific situation, it is best to seek clarification.

Caring, Kindness, Compassion

People respond to being treated kindly and considerately. Use the skills and tools you naturally have, as well as those you have learned in this book. Establish open communication with concerned relations and then make the effort to understand their concerns, their needs and wants, and the motivation behind their upset.

When you can do this, you will remove many obstacles to this problem situation's resolution. Then follow through by focusing on what you can say and do to alleviate their concerns.

Keep in mind that your focus and understanding will eventually be appreciated, if not right away. When you acknowledge other people's concerns you are effectively saying to them: I understand, I care, I respect you and your feelings, I want to help as much as I can. People will remember your efforts in their time of stress and need.

Get help

Sometimes a person or group of people can be overwhelming. It can help immensely to bring another Nurse or a supervisor in to help calm everyone down to the point where you can move ahead with addressing their concerns.

Reiterating: ALWAYS keep your safety and the safety of others paramount. If there is ever any sense of things turning nasty or violent, get help.

Intermediary

Sometimes you do serve as a liaison or intermediary between the Doctor and family members, the patient and family members, and so on. Use your communication skills effectively and keep in mind that 'asking' is always a great tool. It can open up everyone's ability to interrelate on a more congenial level and it gives people a sense of ownership, control, and respect.

The Seven Keys

Questions and concerns? Not sure how to deal with a situation? The "Seven Keys to Understanding and Working with Difficult People," which you will find detailed in Appendix I, serve as a foundation for success with all difficult people issues. With the knowledge you have gained by reading this book, you will have a good feel for how to use these ideas in any problem situation in which you find yourself.

> Self-awareness
>
> Self-worth
>
> Self-Confidence

Self-control

Kindness

Honesty

Positivity

Questions and Ideas for Contemplation

Envision a situation in which a difficult (rude, abrasive, or belligerent) family member is causing you difficulties. Then review ideas in key sections of this book (see Chapters 1, 6, 10, 15, 19 as good general review sections, also Appendix I). Do you feel confident that you will be able to succeed with this difficulty?

Working through several of these types of scenarios can help build your confidence and ability to adjust. Practice will help prepare you for unseen difficulties ahead.

Chapter 22

Working with Authority Figures

"To be great is not to be placed above humanity, ruling others;
but to stand above the partialities and futilities of uniformed
desire, and to rule one's self."

(Spinoza)

The people you work for and with have a marked influence on
how you feel, and hence can affect your overall approach to work
and others. Your relationship with your immediate supervisor and
the Physicians you contact and work with on a daily basis set the
stage for interacting with patients.

Power

However you look at it, Supervisors, Physicians, and other people
in authority positions typically have some type of power and/or
control over our work lives. Power/the perception of power
creates a completely different environment in regard to solving
concerns that may arise that are directly relevant to how we feel
we are treated, communications, general atmosphere, and so on.

You can be successful even with very difficult authority figures,
but it is wise to keep the 'power' issue in mind.

Control

When coupled with the 'power' issue, control takes on a new
perspective when we work with a difficult authority figure. Keep
this important idea in mind:

Difficult people need to feel in control.

When it is your boss, it is a wise idea to figure out ways to let
them have it (or think they have it), while maintaining your own

self-worth, self-confidence, and self-control.

And this Key Idea:

**Control of others is largely an illusion;
self-control is the only true form of control.**

Bosses are People, too

This may be a tough idea to swallow sometimes, but when we can focus on the positive qualities our boss has – and they all do have them – we begin to shift our understanding of them. It can make our relationship with them easier to handle. When we focus on the good qualities of others, the negative stuff will actually become less important and may even become less prevalent. When we focus on the positive qualities of another, we are showing them respect, acknowledgment, and recognition. This will help feed their need for attention, power, and control.

As with all difficult people, focusing on and trying to fulfill their needs and desires can make all the difference in your ability to turn around your relationship with them. Making the effort to understand others often goes a long way toward alleviating personal concerns with them.

You can Learn from them

There is rarely (never?) a difficult person or situation you can't learn something from. Generally the Physicians and Nursing Supervisors you work with have an extensive knowledge base. If you can get around their difficult behaviors and focus on learning things from them, you will set up a different relationship with them that can be positive for both of you.

Also, keep in mind that you can always learn 'what not to do' and 'how not to approach' others from difficult people – not to mention, 'how not to lead.'

Observe

The best tool you have for learning is observation: self-observation, and the understanding you can glean from watching others and how they interact. Take advantage of every situation you are in for personal growth.

The Seven Keys (again!)

Fundamentally you can always return to the basics in your work with any difficult person. Work through your understanding of the "Seven Keys to Understanding and Working with Difficult People: Self-Awareness, Self-Worth, Self-Confidence, Self-Control, Kindness, Honesty, and Positivity." With these Keys as a foundation you will have a solid base upon which to build your interactions with difficult authority figures. [See Appendix I]

Focus on Behaviors

What usually upsets us about an authority figure are things like: how they treat us and others, their overall demeanor, how they communicate, and so on. When you make the attempt to separate the difficult presenting behaviors from the person, you have a chance to succeed. It is far easier to learn how to deal with a difficult behavior than a 'difficult person.'

Intimidation is a frequently used 'tool' of difficult authority figures. You don't have to buy into that just because they are an authority figure. When you don't, and when you can be positive and assertive, they tend to back off their attempts to 'put you in your place.' Bullies don't like to be calmly and professionally challenged. It is not their idea of fun at all. Don't give them the satisfaction by backing off or fighting back. Maintain your professional caring approach regardless of their behavior.

There are always positive ways we can deal with difficult behaviors. As you develop your knowledge, skills, and tools, you will also develop the self-confidence and self-control to be able to handle a wide variety of concerns. Be proactive, solution-oriented, and maintain that positive, calm, caring professional you always intend to be. You will be able to work wonders.

> Author's Note: My book, *Succeeding with Difficult Bosses*, specifically addresses the many issues raised when employees have to work with less than ideal authority figures. If you have had or feel you currently

have difficulties with a person in power over you at work, this would be an excellent book to read. It discusses many specific ideas and scenarios relevant to dealing with difficult authority figures and the concerns they can create in our lives.

Questions and Ideas for Contemplation

Have a difficult boss? Take some time to work out very specifically what it is that is troubling. Some things may be obvious, others more subtle. Write all this out on paper (or type into your computer) in one long 'gripe' session to yourself. Once it is down in some concrete form you will have the basis for which to begin your positive work in solving your concerns with them.

This exercise can be very therapeutic. It is well worth the effort. Be sure to keep your work and notes very private – your eyes only.

Chapter 23

Coworkers

"Interpersonal conflict among Nurses is a significant issue confronting the Nursing profession."

(McKenna, et al, *Journal of Advanced Nursing*, 42(1), 90-96)

Fellow employees who are more or less on the same level as we are can present many difficulties in the work place. Usually these difficulties center around control issues, egos, and perceived slights and differences between people. You can be successful. It all starts with your willingness to take responsibility for yourself, and your ability to step beyond the pettiness of office politics and the games people play.

Over half the participants in a study conducted in New Zealand, "Horizontal violence: experiences of Registered Nurses in their first full year of practice," reported being "undervalued by other Nurses." (McKenna, et al)

Ego

Unfortunately egos often creep into the picture at work. You can be assured that egos are at work if there is:

Blaming

Complaining

Defensiveness

Haughtiness

Rudeness or Abrasive behavior

Put-down, superiority-oriented behavior

In short – any negativity, from others or from you!

Hint: if negativity enters the picture, someone's ego is at work.

Want to fight ego in others and keep an eye on it in yourself?

Practice:

> Kindness
>
> Compassion
>
> Honesty
>
> Professionalism
>
> Self-awareness
>
> And – stay within your own Self-Worth

Differences

The most common cause of difficulties between people is that we are different.

> She may like to do something one way, he another
>
> He is outgoing, she's reserved
>
> Don is concerned with getting things absolutely right; Ed would rather get them done
>
> Alyce likes to follow rules and regulations to the letter, Betty would like some creative flexibility in interpreting guidelines and rules.
>
> And so on – never the twain shall meet.

Differences spice up life and they are one of the most fundamental ways we can learn things from others **if we pay attention!** A free-spirited-sort can learn a great deal from more organized, 'picky' people simply because that is not what they are naturally good at – and vice-versa. Differences can also serve as wake-up calls just when we need them.

Celebrate the differences in others – you can work with them, instead of fighting them!

Irritations

Things that bother us about another person may be the very things we need to pay attention to in ourselves. Perhaps they are things we are not good at. Or perhaps they are things we are really good at and we wish the other person would be good at them too. In either case, we can learn about ourselves and about others by paying attention to irritants in our lives.

Practice patience, understanding, and be willing to help out and support, or at the least accept the differences and foibles of others, rather than fight them.

Be willing to open up and talk about issues with another person. You might be very surprised at what you find out about them. Someone needs to be the positive catalyst – why not you?

YOU are the key

Only you can make a difference. If you are waiting for the other person to change, you will have a long wait. Even if you are RIGHT and they are WRONG, proving it to them or someone else isn't going to make things better. What makes things better in the work place is positivity, which you can spread at every turn and with every person you interact with:

> Compliment others

> Say 'Thank You' a lot

> Appreciate them

> Honor and Recognize them for the good things they do

> Acknowledge them for who they are and what they do bring to the table

> Remember to use the "Seven Keys to Understanding and Working with Difficult People"

> Choose positivity, not negativity

> **"Celebrate what's right with the world."**

> (*National Geographic*)

Another way to look at this is:

> Aren't there already enough people
> 'Celebrating what's wrong with the world'?

Author's Note: My book, *Succeeding with Difficult Coworkers*, specifically addresses the many issues raised when employees have relationships with fellow employees that are concerning. If you have had or feel you currently have difficulties with a colleague, this would be an excellent book to read.

Questions and Ideas for Contemplation

Problems at work? YOU can be the catalyst for change. Yes, it will take some effort and it may take a good bit of time, but isn't it worth it? Your other choice is to blame, complain, whine, point your finger, not take responsibility, wallow in negativity – is this the real you?

Choose wisely.

Chapter 24

Moral and Ethical Issues

"Moral conflict can occur when duties and obligations of health care providers or general guiding ethical principles are unclear...continuing unresolved moral conflicts concerning patient care can have a serious impact on the ability of health care providers to deliver adequate care and influence the amount and type of care that patients receive."

(Jormsri, *Nursing and Health Sciences*, 2004, 6, 217-221)

Nurses have tremendous responsibility in their work. The settings in which you find yourself – hospitals, clinics, home-care, etc. – create many situations that need to be handled delicately, intelligently, and with considerable care. Taking these issues into consideration can help protect you, your patients, and your organization.

Know Your Guidelines

"Making a decision (re. Moral/Ethical conflicts) is often based on a Nurse's perception of the patient's needs, especially when patients lack the capacity to rationally express their own wishes...Nurses have an inherent moral obligation to monitor the care they provide." (Jormsri, 2004).

All businesses are careful about setting guidelines surrounding personnel issues. It is important to become familiar with those of your employer and to stay up-to-date. You should receive information and training. In addition, Human Resources should have materials and other resources available to help keep you informed. It is a good idea to review these types of materials on a regular basis.

I highly recommend open discussions coordinated by Human Resources, your Nursing Program, Supervisor, etc. on Ethical and Moral issues. It is a great way to keep everyone apprised of the latest issues and how they should be handled.

Personal Boundaries

In addition to rules and guidelines established by your organization, it is wise to consider in some depth your own personal boundaries and perspectives on these types of issues. Be sure to:

Know what is important to you, your personal boundaries – what you are willing to accept or not accept (see also Chapter 20, "Sexual and Physical Harassment).

Be willing to stand up for what you believe – Your self-worth and self confidence are key factors in being successful in your profession. If you feel you have to compromise those qualities and values that you feel are the foundation of who you are, you have the right to let others know where your boundaries are.

When you are sensitive to a particular issue or concern it is a good idea to let others know, particularly your supervisor and/or attending Physician. People can be more sensitive to who you are and what your basic beliefs are if they know in advance. It is also respectful to everyone – yourself and others – to be able to share important issues.

Be willing to talk openly about concerns that arise – this is very important, as what may be a powerful issue for you, may not be seen or interpreted that way by someone else, including other people who may be involved directly or indirectly.

Discuss with your supervisor or attending Physician – make sure you are clear about your concerns, and that you are understood. Follow-up if the situation continues. Letting them know up-front that you have strong feelings about a particular issue is essential and helpful to all concerned.

It is a good idea to document specific issues in writing, date, and sign. Send copies to appropriate venues at work: Human Resources, Physician, Supervisor, etc., and keep a copy for your own records.

Seek guidance on issues that you are unclear about or that

raise personal concerns – keeping silent may exacerbate the problem and the earlier in the process you seek help the better.

Be willing to raise issues with whomever is involved. If necessary bring together personnel who may be concerned with the issue, those who can help mediate, those who can provide guidance, anyone who can help resolve the concern.

Be willing to address new issues immediately. Any delay could make it more difficult to deal with if the concern becomes more of an issue.

Take care of yourself and seek support when you are dealing with difficult issues (see next Chapter). These types of concerns can be very stressful and emotionally draining.

Seek help from Human Resources, or personal legal assistance, if you feel it will help.

Considerations

Many moral and ethical issues are not exactly black and white. What becomes important, then, is your ability to understand as much as you can about your own responsibilities, your own personal feelings relevant to the issue, and how others feel about the issue. Here are some things to keep in mind:

Differences – we all look at the world slightly differently – this is especially true in regards to moral and ethical issues. When you are dealing with a concern that is not clear cut, make an effort to understand all the ramifications of the issue:

> Who is involved and how do they feel, what do they think?

> What ideas are impacting this issue – and does everyone understand what they are?

> Have you made your thoughts and feelings understood?

> Can you, or someone else, facilitate discussion about the issue?

> Understand 'the other side' – while you may not agree,

nor ever agree with another person's perspective on the issue, it is wise to make a concerted effort to understand their position and how they feel. This will often open possible directions for compromise toward resolving the concern.

Make every effort to be respectful of others' opinions, even if you do not agree with them. This can also help move things forward, toward an understanding and possible solution. People like to be acknowledged for what they believe, even if you don't completely share those beliefs.

Compromise and Flexibility – often it is possible for people to talk through issues and arrive at a satisfactory middle ground, or at the very least understand each other's position. They can "agree to disagree." Keeping communication channels open is a key factor in resolving moral and ethical concerns.

Communication – people are often reluctant to discuss sensitive issues. You may need to be the catalyst to make this happen. Choosing an appropriate neutral setting, getting interested parties together, setting a format for discussion, being willing to take the lead and open up the proceedings, etc., are things you can do to facilitate an action/solution-driven approach to the concern.

The issue may be very sensitive politically, organizationally, etc. If this is something that needs to be addressed on a more global scale, find out everything you can about the issue and seek guidance from appropriate people and venues at work – Supervisors, Physicians, Human Resources, etc.

Trust

One issue that is often part of difficult concerns and situations at work is our ability to trust others and just as importantly our feelings about whether we are trusted.

Trust is a two-way street and you establish it through your professionalism, your integrity, and your ability to care for others. While you may wish for others to trust you, what is closer to the truth is that in many ways we must earn trust. One of the best way to do that is to trust others.

Suspiciousness, blaming, complaining, whining, backstabbing and similar behaviors can and do quickly undermine the ability of people to function well together and to enjoy their place of work. While these behaviors may be being perpetrated by others, you don't ever want to add to that mix. You can change the dynamics of a workplace by being trustworthy and by giving others a chance – you can establish this type of atmosphere through your own positive communications:

> Being open – surreptitious behavior cannot survive if someone (and then others) keep bringing innuendo and under-handed things/comments out in the open. It works!

> Being honest – blamers, complainers, etc. have less to whine about when people are forthright and honest about everything

> Being positive (and insisting on it within your purview) – negativity doesn't stand much of a chance if you stick to your guns – always.

> Being trustworthy – do what you have said you will do; or let them know why you can't. Nothing is more frustrating to others communication-wise – to patients/clients, your coworkers and staff – than silence about something you can't follow through with. It may be tough sometimes to admit this, but you will create far less ill-will by being open and honest about it. And your integrity and trustworthiness will remain intact.

It really is astonishing how trustworthy people can become when even one person insists on it. You can do this in two key ways:

> Be trustworthy, i.e. open, honest, positive, willing to talk about anything and everything

> Say it – to do so reinforces others' behavior and reminds them what you believe in

>> "I really appreciate your openness and honesty."

>> "I believe in being open about everything."

>> "I really like Alice, she is straightforward and doesn't mince words. She's a trooper."

"Thanks for sharing that with me, Bob. I know it wasn't easy, but we will all enjoy our work around here more when we can share important issues."

Respect

"Respect other people, not because they are wrong, or even because they are right, but because they are human."

(Cogley/Koob)

When we make an effort to respect others for who they are and what they believe, even if what they believe is diametrically opposed to our own beliefs, we can temper most disagreements and conflicts with intelligence and poise. It also speaks to our own integrity – who we are and how we maintain that self in the most difficult of circumstances.

Many issues – moral, ethical, and other life issues – can be dealt with successfully if we maintain our own integrity.

Who are you?

What are you bringing to the equation?

How will that impact others?

Ask yourself these questions when facing difficult concerns.

Questions and Ideas for Contemplation

I would like to be more specific about Moral and Ethical issues, but the possibilities are endless. As recommended in other Chapters, writing down your ideas, feelings, and concerns can be immensely helpful in dealing with difficult issues. Sharing these with a trusted colleague or even being willing to raise an issue in a meeting can also facilitate your own growth and understanding.

Chapter 25

Taking Care of You

"Be your own best Friend."

(Meier)

As a Nursing Professional you have tremendous responsibilities. You have a wide range of things you do and are responsible for, you work with lots of people in many different roles and guises, and you show resiliency through it all. However, we all are affected by stress, over-work, difficulties, and our many responsibilities at work. Taking care of yourself is smart business.

YOU...

You are the most important person in your life. This is not egotistical; it is the simple truth. If you are not at the top of your game, it will affect others. Making sure you are at the best you can be at any given time is your responsibility.

Take time for yourself

It never fails to floor me that otherwise intelligent, dynamic, professional people run about doing their work with little or no consideration for themselves. Not only is it possible to take time for yourself, it is essential –

It is ESSENTIAL that you take time for yourself!
Because if you don't, you will begin to adversely affect others

Ways to take time for yourself

Two minutes – that's one-hundred-and-twenty seconds, in a comfy chair, on a gurney, (Choose a place and make it happen) – with your eyes closed thinking pleasant thoughts

131

Better yet – take five minutes. It's amazing how rejuvenating this can be and YES, if you make the effort, you can find five minutes. [By the way, if you take a seminar with me, I don't accept any excuses you may come up with for not taking care of yourself!]

Even better – take twenty minutes and get some real rest in. Put on a relaxing CD. You probably don't believe there is any way you are going to find that amount of time. [Want to bet? I teach time management, too.]

Imagery meditation – use those two to five to twenty minutes wisely – creating a pleasant scene in your mind to replace all those stresses and worries is very relaxing and rejuvenating. [I like to think of a beautiful lake with animals all around and I walk about petting the deer and rabbits while just drinking all the peacefulness in.]

Take a short walk outside – no cell phones allowed. This is just you and nature. If you take a walk with a colleague/friend, make a rule that you are not allowed to talk about work.

Have a short talk with someone at work about anything but work. Share some pleasant home/family experiences, etc.

Treat yourself: What gives you that extra boost?

> An ice cream cone once a week, or a candy bar?

> A nice bouquet of flowers or a power tool?

> A call to an old friend or close relative to cheer you up?

> Five minutes surfing the web for vacation spots?

Appreciate, Acknowledge, Recognize, and Reward Yourself

Unfortunately we don't always get the appreciation and recognition we deserve. However, make sure you recognize your own hard work:

> See above – treating yourself

> Pat yourself on the back when you do something well, help someone, go the extra mile, and so on.

> Give yourself a small reward when you deserve it – a movie, a long chat with an old friend that evening, etc.

Best bet – appreciate, acknowledge, recognize, reward others at work

Practice random (and sometimes anonymous) acts of kindness - You will feel good as a result. It is great to help others, and it is the best feeling there is

Help others to receive recognition and reward for the good things they do – it keeps up the morale around the office and sets a precedent for others to follow

Help out when someone else is over-worked, stressed, ill, or down-in-the-dumps. Keep it up on a daily basis and over the long haul they might start to reciprocate, too.

Recognize personal concerns

Stay on top of how you feel. When you are stressed, ill, a bit down, get some support and help. Find ways to take it easy, treat yourself, take some time off.

Another very strange phenomenon in the workplace today is that otherwise intelligent, hardworking people refuse to take a day off when they need it. Slogging through a day when you feel terrible can not only be detrimental to your own well-being, it usually is not a wholly positive experience for anyone within your purview in spite of your best efforts.

It goes back to Self-Awareness. The better we know ourselves, the better we can be for others. It's worth paying attention to and thinking about this every day.

Beating yourself up?

Most of us beat ourselves up far too much. While it is tough to turn around self-deprecating behaviors quickly, you can make a major difference if you pay attention to how you treat yourself with your own self-talk.

Take a week and ear-mark it as a time when you are going to make a consistent effort to watch what you say to yourself. As soon as you make any mental statement that says in essence, 'I'm not good enough.' Turn the statement around by saying something positive and self-affirming, "I am good enough."

> "I'm a real loser. I screwed this up again. I'm never going to get things right."

> Rebuttal: "I'm not a loser. I'm very competent and I'm getting better all the time. I'm a really good Nurse, everyone says so. I can do it..."

When we dismiss ourselves, our competencies, our good qualities, we are 'in negativity.' It is much better to be in a more positive space – for ourselves, for those we work with, and especially for those we are serving – our clients – patients.

Talk yourself UP, not d

        o

          w

            n!

You are worth it!

A Close Friend

One of the greatest gifts we can give ourselves is staying in touch with someone we care about. Call up an old, close friend/buddy, 'just because.' And there are always times when it is worth doing because we feel a bit under the weather.

Questions and Ideas for Contemplation

Though the focus of your job and your day at work is helping others, you do need to take care of yourself. I recommend to my clients that they make up a list of little positive things they can do for themselves throughout the day that they can choose from. While they may never use the list per se, the exercise helps them remember things they like and sets the stage for making more positive choices for themselves throughout their workday.

Chapter 26

Making a Difference

Every Day we can make a Positive Difference in someone's life

One of the remarkable things about the Nursing profession is that 'Making a Positive Difference" in people's lives is the essence of your profession. The question then becomes one of 'How can you make the most of this opportunity?'

> Author's Note: As a writer, motivational speaker, executive and personal coach, and business seminar presenter, I hope to have a positive influence on people's lives, i.e. that I am 'of service' to others. However, often many days go by where my only contact with people is when I get up from my writing and pass someone while walking the dog, or when I go to the store and interact with a clerk, when I speak with someone on the phone, or when I answer e-mails. Plus the very important and precious time spent with my wife before and after her long work days.

The point?

Each of those moments with another person are opportunities to make a positive difference or to make something else.

Though your profession is centered around making a positive difference in the lives of others, truly "Making a Difference," means stepping it up a notch from something that is 'required' to something that is in your heart.

Every day you can make a difference to:

Your patients

Their families and loved ones

Physicians

Your Supervisor(s)

Staff at work

Colleagues

Your own family and friends

Acquaintances

Strangers you meet

Anyone and everyone you have any contact with

Ask yourself these questions

How do you want them to see you?

Who is the true you that you want to bring forth in those moments of time you are with others – patients, supervisors, Physicians, coworkers, friends, relatives, strangers...?

In what ways can you make a difference, a truly positive difference, in their lives? You may only have a second or two – can you do it?

Here's a little true story

A few years ago near the town where I lived, often when I drove down a certain road I would pass an older fellow I began to refer to as 'the Wavy Guy.' 'Wavy Guy' would take long walks along this road, my guess is twice a day, because I passed him quite frequently, and he always waved at every car, truck, SUV, etc., that passed. He coupled that wave with a big smile.

The cool thing about it was that it was infectious because you could tell he was sincere and he enjoyed it. Maybe this guy's always positive approach to others infected me, too, because I often think of him when I think of the small things we can do to make a difference with others.

After awhile, I began to play a little game with myself. I would challenge myself to spot the old fella before he saw me in my truck and I would wave enthusiastically first. I don't know if he was aware of my 'game,' but I think we both had some fun waving at each other and it is that kind of fun that IS infectious.

You carry that with you for the rest of your day and when you feel good it does affect and often, infect, others.

In short – find ways to 'wave' at people every day. There are many things we can do to 'make a difference' at work, at home, and in the world at large. You, as Nurses, are in the unique position where you can make it your mission because, in reality, it is part of your job.

Speaking from experience, there is no feeling quite like making a positive difference in someone else's life.

The problem

Are you over-worked? Taken for granted by patients, supervisors, Physicians? Underpaid? Stressed? Working too long shifts? Getting 'beat-up' on a regular basis? Beating yourself up on a regular basis?

Some or all of the above could be true – can you raise yourself above these and still 'make a difference?'

You can if you pay attention – if you remind yourself –
if you DO make it part of your mission for yourself and others.

There are a myriad of ways, often very subtle ways, we can make a positive difference with/for others. Sometimes it is the simple things that have the most impact and the things that we might think last about doing.

Also, keep in mind that everything you do at work affects everyone at work – including your patients – because it all comes back to how you feel. Here are a few ideas below, but take some time to generate your own mental (or written) list of things you can do to make a difference. I guarantee you will be glad you did:

Give lots of sincere, small compliments (you don't have to wait for major successes)

Say 'Thank you' at every opportunity

Touch people's lives in some small way

Do something for them even if it's not 'your job'

> Support them when they need it
>
> Be a good listener (especially without judgment or interruption)
>
> Give little gifts (even a tiny flower found in the parking lot can elicit a smile)

Smile a lot!

Be the opposite of negative – always!

Say it! Sometimes sharing a positive thought, idea, or response can work wonders.

Send an upbeat (rather than 'business') e-mail (it can take five or ten seconds)

Tell someone you appreciate them

Tell someone you care. Better yet – show it!

Dream a little, use your imagination, jump on opportunities that present themselves – have some fun with this.

YOU can make the most amazing difference at work REGARDLESS of how other people are. You can! I've seen it happen; I've done it. You don't have to be over-the-top, the most infectious positive personality around; you have to be:

> The TRUE you – that person that you sincerely believe in bringing into the world. [See exercise in Chapter 9]
>
> You also have to remind yourself every day that you can make a difference.
>
> Yes, it will take some time
>
> It will take perseverance
>
> It will take caring for yourself, so you bring the best of you to others
>
> It will take your willingness to CARE about and for others.

Best to all of you in an Honorable and Caring Profession,

Joe Koob

Appendix I

The Seven Keys to Being Successful with Difficult People

These seven key ideas are the backbone of the materials presented throughout the Difficultpeople.org website. They have been developed by Dr. Koob through his extensive experience and study relevant to difficult people and difficult situations. As you begin to understand more and more about dealing successfully with difficult people come back to these Key Ideas. You will find they offer a tremendous amount of insight and support.

The "Seven Keys to being Successful with Difficult People" came about through the ongoing development of literature available at www.difficultpeople.org – a web site dedicated to "Understanding and Working with Difficult People." As you work on your understanding and strengths in these important areas you will notice a marked difference and improvement in how you perceive 'difficult' people you interact with and how you handle their 'difficult' interpersonal behaviors.

These "Seven Keys" are all centered in your attitude about yourself and others

Working successfully with other people centers around how we feel about ourselves. Their 'stuff' has a direct effect on how they interact with us but does not have to affect how we feel or go about our own work. When we can step beyond their problems and live our life to the fullest and make the most of our work on OUR terms, we have learned to truly be in control.

Self-awareness

Self-worth

Self-Confidence

Self-Control

Honesty

Kindness

Positivity

Self-awareness

Self-awareness tops this list because it is fundamental to all the other ideas. When we begin to understand ourselves better, we can make better choices, and we strengthen our self-worth, self-confidence, and self-control. There is no better tool available for you to help build your foundation for dealing effectively and positively with others.

Working on your self-awareness pays big dividends. It is helpful to start this process by reading more extensive materials on how to develop these skills. [See *Understanding and Working with Difficult People*; *Me! A Difficult Person?* and *A Perfect Day: Guide for a Better Life (Koob, J.)*]

Self-worth

Self-worth is how we value ourselves. It has nothing to do with ego – placing ourselves above others. It has to do with who we truly believe ourselves to be and how we bring that belief to the world. It has to do with understanding our most fundamental values – who we would most like to be with others.

Self-confidence

As we develop our self-worth our self-confidence improves. Many of the difficulties we have with other people are affected a great deal by our inability to maintain a confident and positive demeanor when we are with them. You can be assured that if you are getting upset, defensive, depressed, etc. that your confidence is taking a hit.

Self-confident people approach others from an assertive stance. Assertiveness is being able to accept yourself in an interaction with another person regardless of their behavior. It does take practice and self-awareness.

Self-control

Control of other people is an illusion. It is an illusion that drives difficult people to their difficult behaviors. To be successful with difficult people our only recourse is **self-control**. We are not out to control them, only our own feelings, thoughts, and responses to their difficult behaviors. When we are in control, they almost always don't have any choice but to change their negative behavior when interacting with us.

No one can control our lives without our permission! We always have positive choices we can make. Sometimes they are difficult to understand or to see. Practice in self-awareness, awareness and understanding of others, and in developing our self-worth and self-confidence can make all the difference.

Honesty

Honesty means being honest with ourselves (more self-awareness!) and being **kindly** honest with others.

You always have a right to be honest with others and there are ALWAYS positive, assertive ways to do that.

Kindness

Every interaction we have with other people has the opportunity for us to be kind, or to be something else. Practicing kindness, especially in the face of difficult behavior, pays huge dividends. Try it! You will be pleasantly surprised.

It can be really tough to be kind and compassionate in the face of a very disagreeable, inflexible person. Try to keep in mind that this difficult person is a child of the universe no less than you. Whatever 'stuff,' past and current, has them where they currently are, is perhaps quite unfortunate, for you, and especially for them. You may be able to make a positive difference to their existence, even if it is only for a short time. And you may very well be the catalyst that helps them start to turn their life around.

Positivity

This can be summed up in one of Dr. Koob's favorite sayings:

Negativity breeds Negativity

Positivity Breeds Positivity

Choose Wisely

Another way to say this is:

Negativity NEVER helps!

These are worth thinking about!

Appendix II

Difficultpeople.org Books

Annotated Bibliography

Understanding and Working with Difficult People

We believe this book presents the most comprehensive material available about being successful with difficult people. This book is designed to be a practical, accessible introduction to the very broad topic of dealing with difficult people/difficult behaviors. Since every difficult situation is different, the focus here will be on building a basic understanding of how you interact with difficult people, what makes difficult people tick, and the most fundamental skills you can bring to the table to help change these encounters for the better.

ME! A Difficult Person?

This is second of our signature books. This book focuses on learning more about yourself. Most of us are occasionally difficult or seen as difficult by others. This may simply be a matter of different perspectives, or it may mean that we have some inner work to do. This course is concerned with understanding more about how you come across to others, and understanding more about who you are as a person. It is also concerned with self-improvement – making changes that will help make your interactions with others significantly better, and that will bring you more peace, comfort, and joy in your life.

Difficult Spouses? Improving and Saving Your Relationship with Your Significant Other

Are you having difficulties in your current relationship? Facing a divorce? Newly divorced and trying to understand what happened and what you could have done about it? We feel this book has value not only for couples who are simply having difficulties in their relationships with their significant others; those facing divorce, recently divorced couples; and for people entering new relationships. The focus is on developing the knowledge, skills, and tools to help your relationship be successful.

Dealing with Difficult Strangers

Being successful in difficult situations with strangers is all about what you can bring to the situation. You will find a tremendous amount of useful information and skills included in this book that can make a significant difference in how you approach difficult strangers, how you feel as a result of these difficult encounters, and how you can emerge without a negative experience having ruined your day.

Succeeding with Difficult Professors (and Tough Courses)

A course for college students at all levels. What you need to know to make the most of your college career. This course has two main sections: "Getting along with Difficult Professors," and "Succeeding in Tough Classes." The first section will discuss ideas and skills you can use to get through personal difficulties with professors. The second section will focus on techniques, study skills, and approaches that will help you get the grades you want.

Guiding Children

Guiding and working with children is on the mind of every parent. This book focuses on skills and tools to help you as a parent provide the best possible environment for your child's development by avoiding difficulties through intelligent upbringing. This book is not only about helping you to guide your children through concerns that arise, but it is even more about enjoying your children. They do grow up, much faster than we expect. Take advantage of the tremendous joy they can bring into your life and the vast understanding of life that they provide. You will be glad you did.

Business Trilogy: Dealing with Change

Difficult Situations - Dealing with Change

Difficult situations can certainly produce a great deal of angst and as a result, difficult people. From my own long personal experience, I know that when things are tough, I can get much more difficult than normal. Those are the times when I know I need to deal with my own stuff.

Honoring Work and Life: 99 Words for Leaders to Live By

This book provides a foundation of key ideas that focus on Leadership (and Personal) qualities, attributes, and behaviors that honor not only our work but our life. It is my firm belief that true leaders work to serve their fellow employees, their team, their company, their customers, as well as their families and friends. This is about understanding and working on those attributes that make great leaders.

Leaders Managing Change

Leaders Managing Change is about understanding and dealing with the ongoing stresses of constant change in the business world today, but most importantly it is about leadership. When I thought about the concerns that are a regular part of high turnover rates, leadership changes, acquisitions and mergers, and the myriad of other transitions businesses face today, the focus came down to leadership. Good leaders get things done. This book focuses on knowledgeable leadership, i.e. what you need to know to help you deal with change as a leader. It presumes you are already inspired, good, intelligent, and practical. This book is about making a difference.

Dealing with Difficult Customers

(for Employees, Companies, and Customer Service Personnel)

This book is all about putting the gamut of customer relations and interactions into a perspective that is workable, livable, and supports you, the customer contact person, throughout.

While many businesses do provide extensive customer relations training, the focus is often fairly one way – aimed at keeping business. We present you with extensive insight and knowledge about the customer's perspective, what you need to know as a company representative to fulfill your job, the internal and external support you need, and the tools and skills to communicate effectively with difficult customers.

Business Trilogy: Succeeding at Work

Dealing with Difficult Coworkers

This work is one that based on my research is a needed addition to the difficult people literature. There are a number of books available that discuss difficult people in the workplace, but do not focus specifically on coworkers. There are different dynamics between bosses and employees, employees and their peers, and employees with their bosses. The emphasis here is on helping people solve the difficulties they have at work with someone who is relatively speaking a 'coworker,' or 'colleague,' in other words, someone whose 'rank' or 'job' is roughly on the same level as theirs.

Succeeding with Difficult Bosses

Have a tough boss? This is a practical, in-the-trenches approach to succeeding with a difficult authority figure – a (how to) book for one of your most important relationships at work.

Managing Difficult Employees

In Production

Caring for Difficult Patients: A Guide for Nursing Professionals

I believe that the Nursing profession is one of the most admired in America. We think of Nurses as professional: that is, they have a knowledge base and skill set that is unique and valued – the quality of their work is important to them; and we think of Nurses as people who care about their patients – they are concerned with our well-being when we are under their care. These considerations are the focal point for discussing how to best deal with difficult patients.

Bibliography

Articles & Books

Nursing

Benner, P. & Wrubel, J., *The primacy of caring: Stress and coping in health and illness.* Menlo Park, CA: Addison-Wesley, 1988.

Farrell, Gerald A., "Aggression in clinical settings: Nurses' views – a follow-up study", *Journal of Advanced Nursing,* 1999; 29(3): 532-541.

Farrell, Gerald A., "From Tall poppies to squashed weeds: why don't Nurses pull together more?" *Journal of Advanced Nursing,* 2001; 35(1): 26-33.

Freedman, Melanie, Dealing effectively with Difficult People, *Nursing,* 1993; 97-102.

Jormsri, Pantip, "Moral conflict and collaborative mode as moral conflict resolution in health care," *Nursing and Health Sciences,* 2004; 6: 217-221.

Koob, P.B., *The Curriculum Revolution in Practice: A Heideggeruan Hermeneutical Analysis of the Lived Experience of Women Nurse Educators. Dissertation,* 1996.

McKenna, Smith, Poole, and Cloverdale, "Horizontal Violence: experiences of Registered Nurses in their first year of practice," *Journal of Advanced Nursing,* 2003; 42 (1): 90-96.

Orr, Robert D., "Methods of Conflict Resolution at the Bedside," *ajob,* Fall 2001; Vol.1, #4: 45-46.

Pointon, Clare, "Conflict Resolution – can it really work?" *Counseling & Psychotherapy Journal,* Feb. 2005; Vo. 16,(1).

Porter-O'Grady, Tim, "Constructing a Conflict Resolution Program for Health Care," *Health Care Manage Rev,* 2004; 29(4): 278-283.

Santamaria, N., "The Difficult Patient Stress Scale: a new instrument to measure interpersonal stress in Nursing," *Australian Journal of Advanced Nursing*, 1995-1996; 13(2): 22-29.

Santamaria, N., "The relationship between Nurses' personality and stress levels reported when caring for interpersonally difficult patients," *Australian Journal of Advanced Nursing*, 2000-2001, 18(2): 20-26.

Seeman, Bruce T., "For Nurses, a touchy issue: Sexual harassment by patients adds to heavy career stress," Newhouse News Service, *The Ann Arbor News*, 20 Dec 2005.

Skjorshammer, Morten, "Physician in Conflict: A Survey Study of Individual and Work-related Characteristics," *Scandinavian Journal of Caring Science*, 1999; 212-216.

Tanner, P., Reflections of the curriculum revolution. *Journal of Nursing Education*, 1990, 29(7). 295-299.

Difficult People Materials

Axelrod, A and Holtje, J., *201 Ways to Deal with Difficult People*, McGraw-Hill, New York, 1997.

Bell, A. and Smith, D., *Winning with Difficult People*, Barron's, New York, 1997

Bramson, Robert M., *Coping with Difficult Bosses*, Fireside, New York, 1992.

Bramson, Robert M., *Coping with Difficult People*, Anchor Press, New York, 1981.

Braunstein, Barbara, *How to Deal with Difficult People*, Skillpath Publications, Mission, KS, 1994. [Tapes]

Brinkman, R. and Kirschner, R., *Dealing with People You Can't Stand*, McGraw-Hill, New York, 1994.

Carter, Jay, *Nasty Bosses: How to STOP BEING HURT by them without stooping to THEIR level*, McGraw-Hill, New York, 2004.

Case, Gary and Rhoades-Baum, *How to Handle Difficult Customers*, Help Deck Institute, Colorado Springs, 1994.

Cava, Roberta, *Dealing with Difficult People: How to Deal with Nasty Customers, Demanding Bosses and Annoying Co-workers*, Firefly Books, Buffalo, NY, 2004.

Cava, Roberta, *difficult people: How to Deal with Impossible clients, Bosses, and Employees*, Firefly Books, Buffalo, NY, 1990.

Cavaiola, A. And Lavender, N., *Toxic Coworkers: How to Deal with Dysfunctional People on the Job*, New Harbinger Publications, Oakland, CA, 2000.

Costello, Andrew, *How to Deal with Difficult People*, Ligori Publications, Liguri, MI, 1980.

Crowe, Sandra, *Since Strangling Isn't An Option*, Perigee, New York, 1999.

Diehm, William, *How to Get Along with Difficult People*, Broadman Press, Nashville, 1992.

Felder, Leonard, *Does Someone Treat You Badly? How to Handle Brutal Bosses, Crazy Coworkers...and Anyone Else Who Drives You Nuts*, Berkley Books, NY, 1993.

First, Michael, Ed., *Diagnostic and Statistical Manual for Mental Disorders*, 4th Edition, American Psychiatric Asso.,Washington, 1994.

Friedman, Paul, *How to Deal with Difficult People*, SkillPath Publications, Mission, KS, 1994.

Gill, Lucy, *How to Work with Just About Anyone*, Fireside, New York, 1999.

Griswold, Bob, *Coping with Difficult and Negative People and Personal Magnetism*, Effective Learning Systems, Inc., Edina, MN. [Tape]

Holloway, Andy, "Bad Boss Blues," *Canadian Business*, 24 Oct 2004.

Hoover, John, *How to Work for an Idiot: Survive & Thrive Without Killing Your Boss*, Career Press, Princeton, NJ, 2004.

Jones, Katina, *Succeeding with Difficult People*, Longmeadow Press, Stamford, CT, 1992.

Keating, Charles, *Dealing with Difficult People*, Paulist Press, New York, 1984.

Littauer, Florence, *How to Get Along with Difficult People*, Harvest House, Eugene, 1984.

Lloyd, Ken, *Jerks at Work: How to Deal with People Problems and Problem People*, Career Press, Franklin Lakes, NJ, 1999

Lundin, W. and Lundin, J., *When Smart People Work for Dumb Bosses: How to Survive in a Crazy and Dysfunctional Workplace*, McGraw-Hill, New York, 1998.

Markham, Ursula, *How to deal with Difficult people*, Thorsons, London, 1993.

Meier, Paul, *Don't Let Jerks Get the Best of You: Advice for Dealing with Difficult People*, Thomas Nelson, Nashville, 1993.

Namie, G. and Namie, R., *the Bully at Work*, Sourcebooks, Inc., Naperville, IL, 2000.

Osbourne, Christina, *Dealing with Difficult People*, DK, London, 2002.

Oxman, Murray, *The How to Easily Handle Difficult People, Success Without Stress*, Morro Bay, CA, 1997.

Perkins, Betty, *Lion Taming: The Courage to Deal with Difficult People Including Yourself*, Tzedakah Publications, Scramento, 1995.

Rosen, Mark, *Thank You for Being Such A Pain: Spiritual Guidance for Dealing with Difficult People*, Three Rivers Press, New York, 1998.

Segal, Judith, *Getting Them to See It Your Way: Dealing with Difficult and Challenging People*, Lowell House, Los Angeles, 2000.

Solomon, Muriel, *Working with Difficult People*, Prentice Hall, Englewood Cliffs,1990.

Toropov, Brandon, *The Complete Idiot's Guide to Getting Along with Difficult People*, Alpha Books, New York, 1997.

Toropov, Brandon, *Manager's Guide to Dealing with Difficult People*, Prentice Hall, Paramus, NJ, 1997.

Turecki, Stanley, *The Difficult Child*, Bantam Books, NY, 1989.

Weiner, David L., *Power Freaks: Dealing with Them in the Workplace or Anywhere*, Prometheus Books, Amherst, New York, 2002

Weiss, Donald, *How to Deal with Difficult People*, Amacon, New York, 1987.

Recommended Readings

Dewey, John, *Democracy and Education*, Norwood Press, Norwood, MA, 1916.

Dewey, John, *Education and Experience*, Kappa Delta Pi Publications, Macmillian, New York, 1938.

Dyer, Wayne, *Pulling Your Own Strings*, Funk and Wagnalls, New York, 1978.

Dyer, Wayne, *Your Erroneous Zones*, Funk and Wagnalls, New York, 1976.

Dyer, Wayne, *Your Sacred Self*, Harper, New York, 1995.

Guraik, David B., Editor, *Webster's New World Dictionary*, World Publishing, New York, 1972.

Heinlein, Robert, *Time Enough for Love*, New English Library, New York, 1974.

Hesse, Hermann, *Narcissus and Goldmund*, Bantam, New York, 1971.

James, M, and Jongeward, D. *Born to Win*, Addison-Wesley, 1971.

Koob, Joseph, *A Perfect Day: Guide for A Better Life*, NEJS Publications, Lawton, OK, 1998.

Parrott, Thomas Marc, Ed., *Shakespeare: Twenty-three Plays and the Sonnets*, Charles Scribner's Sons, Washington, D.C., 1938.

Pirsig, Robert, *Zen and the Art of Motorcycle Maintenance*, Bantam, New York, 1980.

Rand, Ayn, *Atlas Shrugged*, Signet Books, New York, 1957.

Redman, Ben Ray, Editor, *The Portable Voltaire*, Viking Press, New York, 1949.

Books and other works on Change and Leadership

Bolles, Richard N., *What Color is Your Parachute?* Ten Speed Press, Berkeley, CA, 1987.

Bridges, William, *Managing Transitions: Making the Most of Change*, Perseus Books, Cambridge, 1991.

Bridges, William, *Transitions: Making Sense of Life's Changes*, Perseus Books, Cambridge, 1980.

Buckingham, Marcus, & Coffman, Curt, *First, Break All the Rules: What the World's Greatest Managers Do Differently*, Simon and Schuster, New York, 1999.

Collins, J., and Porras, J., *Built to Last: Successful Habits of Visionary Companies*, Harper Business, NY, 2001.

Collins, Jim, *Good TO Great: Why Some Companies Make the Leap...and Others Don't*, Harper Business, NY, 2001.

Cooper, Robert and Sawaf, Ayman, *Executive EQ: Emotional Intelligence in Leadership & Organizations*, Grisset/Putnam, New York, 1996.

Crane, Thomas, *The Heart of Coaching*, FTA Press, San Diego, 1998.

Deits, Bob, Life *After Loss: A Personal Guide Dealing with Death, Divorce, Job Change and Relocation*, Fisher Books, Tucson, 1988.

Dominhguez, Linda R., *How to Shine at Work*, McGraw Hill, 2003.

Drucker, Peter F., *Managing in a Time of Great Change*, Truman Talley Books, NY, 1995.

Evard, Beth L. And Gipple, Craig A., *Managing Business Change for Dummies*, Hungry Minds, Inc., NY, 2001.

Farson, Richard and Keyes, Ralph, *Whoever Makes the Most Mistakes Wins: The Paradox of Innovation*, Free Press, NY, 2002.

Fortgang, Laura Berman, *Take Yourself to the Top: The Secrets of America's #1 Career Coach*, Warner Books, New York, 1998.

Gates, Bill, *Business @ the Speed of Thought: Succeeding in the Digital Economy*, Warner Books, New York, 1999.

Gerstner, Jr., Louis, V, *Who Says Elephants Can't Dance? Leading a Great Enterprise Through Dramatic Change*, HarperBusiness, New York, 2002.

Going Through Bereavement–When a loved one dies, Langeland Memorial Chapel, Kalamazoo, MI.

Grieve, Bradly T., *The Blue Day Book: A Lesson in Cheering Yourself Up*, Andrews McMeel Publishing, Kansas City, 2000.

Goldratt, Eliyahu M., *Critical Chain*, North River Press, Great Barrington, MA, 1997.

Hammer, Michael and Champy, James, *Reengineering the Corporation: A Manifesto for Business Revolution, HarperBusiness*, New York, 1993.

Hoffer, Eric, *The Ordeal of Change*, Harper & Row, NY, 1952.

Jeffreys, J. Shep. *Coping with Workplace Change: Dealing with Loss and Grief*, Crisp Productions, Menlo Park, CA, 1995.

Johnson, Spencer, *Who Moved My Cheese*, G. P. Putnam, New York, 1998.

Kanter, Rosabeth Moss, *The Change Masters: Innovation & Entrepreneurship in the American Corporation*, Simon & Schuster, New York, 1983.

Kelley, Robert, *How to be a Star at Work: Nine Breakthrough Strategies You Need to Succeed*, Random House, New York, 1998.

Koob, Joseph E. II, *Difficult Situations: Dealing with Change*, NEJS Publications, Saline, MI, 2004.

Kotter, John P, *Leading Change*, Harvard Business School Press, Boston, 1996.

Kotter, John P, *The Leadership Factor*, Free Press, New York, 1988.

Kouzes, J. and Posner, B., *Credibility: How Leaders Gain and Lose it; Why People Demand it*, Jossey-Bass Publishers, San Francisco, 1993.

Kuster, Elizabeth, *Exorcising Your Ex*, Fireside, New York, 1996.

Leonard, George, *Mastery: The Keys to Success and Long-term Fulfillment*, Plume, NY 1992.

Lunden, Joan, and Cagan, Andrea, *A Bend in the Road is Not the End of the Road,* William Morrow, New York, 1998.

Maxwell, John C., *The 21 Indispensible Qualities of Leadership: Becoming the Person Others Will Want to Follow*, Thomas Nelson Publishers, Nashville, 1999.

Maxwell, John C., *The 17 Indisputable Laws of Teamwork: Embrace them and Empower Your Team*, Thomas Nelson Publishers, Nashville, 2001.

Maxwell, John C., *21 Irrefutable Laws of Leadership*, Thomas Nelson, Inc., Nashville, 1998.

Milwid, Beth, *Working With Men: Professional Women Talk About Power, Sexuality, and Ethics*, Beyond Words, Kingsport, TN, 1990.

McKay, Harvey, *Swim with the Sharks: Without Being Eaten Alive*, William Morrow Co., New York, 1988.

Messer, Bonnie J., *Dealing with Change,* Abington Press, 1996.

Montalbo, Thomas, *The Power of Eloquence: Magic Key to Success in Public Speaking*, Prentive-Hall, Englewood Cliffs, N.J., 1984.

Pasternack, Bruce and Viscio, Albert, *The Centerless Corporation: A New Model for Transforming Your Organization for Growth and Prosperity*, Fireside, New York, 1998.

Peters, Tom, *The Circle of Innovation: You Can't Shrink Your Way to Greatnness*, Vintage Books, New York, 1999.

Peters, Tom, *Liberation Management: Necessary Disorganization for the Nanosecond Nineties*, Faucett Columbine, New York, 1992.

Peters, Tom, and Waterman, Robert, *In Search of Excellence: Lessons from America's Best-Run Companies*, Harper & Row, New York, 1982.

Peters, Tom, and Austin, Nancy, *A Passion for Excellence: The Leadership Difference*, Random House, New York, 1985.

Peters, Tom, *The Pursuit of WOW! Every Person's Guide to Topsy-Turvy Times*, Vintage Books, New York, 1994.

Peters, Tom, *Professional Service Firm 50: Fifty Ways to Transform Your "Department" into a Professional Service Firm whose Trademarks are Passion and Excellence*, Alfred A. Knopf, 1999.

Peters, Tom, *Re-imagine! Business Excellence in a Disruptive Age*, DK, London, 2003.

Peters, Tom, *Thriving on Chaos: Handbook for a Management Revolution*, Alfred Knopf, New York, 1987

Popcorn, Faith, *EVEolutuon: The Eight Truths of Marketing to Women*, Hyperion Books, 2001.

Smith, Hyrum W. The *10 Natural Laws of Successful Time and Life Management: Proven Strategies for Increased Productivity and Inner Peace*, Warner Books, New York, 1994.

Talbot, Kay, *The Ten Biggest Myths About Grief*, Abbey Press, St. Meinrad, IN, 2000.

Waterman, Robert H., Jr., *The Renewal Factor: How The Best Get And Keep The Competitive Edge*, Bantam, New York, 1986.

Whitmore, John, *Coaching for Performance*, Nicholas Brealey Publishing, London, 1999.

LaVergne, TN USA
31 August 2010
195343LV00004B/105/A